"COME AND GET YOUR BEER AND BENZEDRINE!"

—FROM "ON THAT GREAT COME AND GET IT DAY,"
FINIAN'S RAINBOW BY YIP HARBURG

SPEED-SPEED-SPEEDFREAK

A FAST HISTORY OF AMPHETAMINE ● BY MICK FARREN

FERAL HOUSE

TABLE OF CONTENTS

The band had graduated
from pills to glass ampoules of pure liq-
uid methedrine. The running gag among the
musicians and roadies was that the only clinical
use for the stuff, aside from fueling a ramshackle rock
& roll band from one performance hellhole to the next,
was to revive patients who had clinically died on an
operating table. We took a certain suicidally romantic
pride in our advanced substance abuse—it was, after
all, the late 1960s. We might not play as well or be
as popular as The Who, but there was a good chance
we were taking quite as much speed as they were, and
we figured that had to count for something. Some band
members injected the drug, others, the ones with a pho-
bic dislike of needles, simply cracked open the neck of the
ampoule and poured it into a Coca-Cola or a Pepsi...

—MICK FARREN ON THE DEVIANTS

A DRUG IN SEARCH OF A FUNCTION

WHEN BASIC AMPHETAMINE WAS FIRST SYNTHESIZED in 1887 by the Romanian chemist Lazar Edeleanu, working at the University of Berlin, no one was thinking about madness, death, or any combination of the two. The hope was that this new compound would prove an easily manufactured and more efficient bronchodilator for asthmatics than the drug ephedrine, which had been isolated from the plant ma huang that same year by Nagayoshi Nagai in Japan. Edeleanu dubbed his creation "phenylisopropylamine," but later switched its name to alpha-methylphenethylamine which was quickly shortened to the more pronounceable amphetamine. (As in alpha-methylphenethylamine.)

From the very start, amphetamine proved itself to be a drug in search of a function. It had proved disappointing as an asthma cure, but it showed a quite amazing range of side effects. Test subjects exhibited alertness, euphoria, heightened physical energy, and prolonged stamina. In early tests, it enhanced concentration, caused rapid and volatile verbalization, boosted confidence, and increased social responsiveness. Other effects of the drug included decreased appetite, and a noticeable enhancement of the sex drive and sexual response in both men and women. When, again in Japan, in 1919, the related but far more powerful crystallized methamphetamine was synthesized by a research team led by Akira Ogata (via reduction of ephedrine using red phosphorus and iodine), commercial uses still could not be found, but it was noted that the same powerful side effects observed with the original amphetamine were even more pronounced in this advanced variation.

At that point, the research on amphetamine was shelved, and it wasn't until 1927 that pioneer psychopharmacologist Gordon Alles resynthesized the drug, still seeking a substitute for the asthma cure ephedrine, but, again, it failed to fulfill its intended purpose. Although to continue research on a drug without any immediate specific therapeutic goal is common in today's pharmaceutical industry, such work was simply considered a waste of time and laboratory space in the early twentieth century. Alles had, however, discovered that amphetamine could be produced in a volatile form that lent itself to packaging as an inhaler. This attracted the attention of the corporate pharmaceutical giant Smith, Kline & French (SK&F), who decided that amphetamine could be profitably marketed as a means of relief for a whole variety of ailments. In 1932, the Benzedrine inhaler was launched in drugstores in the United States, and was both prescribed by accommodating physicians, and sold over the counter, first as a general treatment for respiratory problems, then within less than three years, for relief of more than 39 medical conditions ranging from hiccups to schizophrenia.

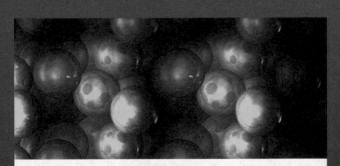

THE ∫CIENCE OF ∫PEED

AMPHETAMINES release stores of norepinephrine and dopamine from nerve endings by converting the respective molecular transporters into open channels. Amphetamine also releases stores of serotonin from synaptic vesicles when taken in relatively high doses. This effect is more pronounced in methamphetamine use. Amphetamines also prevent the monoamine transporters for dopamine and norepinephrine from recycling them (called reuptake inhibition), which leads to increased amounts of dopamine and norepinephrine in synaptic clefts. These combined effects rapidly increase the concentrations of the respective neurotransmitters in the synaptic cleft, which promotes nerve impulse transmission in neurons that have those receptors. ●

WHILE SMITH, KLINE & FRENCH AND THE MEDICAL profession were extolling the virtues of Benzedrine, a section of the ever ingenious public-at-large quickly discovered that the inhalers had an equally extensive nonmedical potential—essentially the range of side effects first observed by the researchers Edeleanu and Nagai—and began to devise ingenious ways to exploit them. The abuse of Benzedrine inhalers required only minimal cunning. The inhaler was a tube about the size of a fat cigarette, a hard case containing either a paper strip or cotton ball saturated in Benzedrine. All this first generation of speedfreaks needed to do was to crack open the casing of the inhaler, and swallow the contents, rolling the paper or cotton into small balls and washing them down with coffee, a soft drink, or alcohol. In 1937, Smith, Kline & French released a pill form of Benzedrine, and "bennies," as instant street slang nicknamed them, became the new recreational drug.

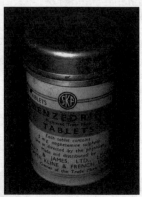

The use of both the pills and inhalers was rapidly adopted on all levels of society. In addition to the usual drug culture lowlifes—the zoot suiters, jazz musicians, strippers, hookers, and petty criminals who might be expected to dunk the contents of a Benzedrine inhaler in their all-night coffee, college kids resorted to them when cramming for exams, or just to party. Long-distance drivers used them to stay awake at the wheel, while factory workers on the newly introduced production lines used bennies to help them work double shifts. Whispered rumors also circulated about the use of Benzedrine as a performance enhancement in professional sports, and doubtless its radical effects on sexual stamina and creativity had also been noted. Back in the pre-Kinsey 1930s, no one wrote openly about the ins and outs of sex and sexual responses except on the level of smudged, cheapo print porn like the time-honored Tijuana Bibles in which bennies are now and then mentioned.

The bizarre paradox, however, was that Benzedrine in particular and amphetamine in general were close to being an exact chemical analogue of traditional American virtues—stamina, dedication, hard work, endurance, and the willingness to repeat mindless actions for hours on end. This fact was not ignored by capitalists and captains of industry. Far from discouraging drug use on the factory floor, a number of industrialists—Henry Ford reputedly among them—studied, at least in theory, the effects that the distribution of amphetamines to the labor force might have on the equation between manpower and productivity in manufacturing industries. A drug that would narrow the machine operator's focus, and make him or her more at one with their machine had to be good for any business from the mighty General Motors to the smallest and most sweaty of garment industry sweatshops.

Meanwhile the old-time Hollywood studio bosses like Harry Cohen and Louis B. Mayer didn't bother to conduct studies. They didn't even hesitate. They saw amphetamine as a chemical tool that could reduce the budgets on their movies, and they immediately put it to use. They went right ahead and fed speed to their performers to keep them animated on camera during extended shoots. (Or, in some cases, to cure monumental movie star hangovers.) Child actors seem to have been par-

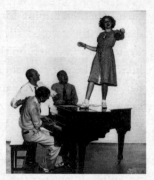

JUDY GARLAND AT 16

ticular targets of this chemical talent enhancement. Both Judy Garland and Mickey Rooney have made no secret of how they were constantly given speed in order to make it through grueling 12- or 14-hour, all-singing, all-dancing shoots. The Judy Garland entry on the Internet Movie Database is totally blunt in its Garland biography: "The same studio that made her a star unwittingly made her a drug addict, providing her with amphetamines to keep her energy level high and her weight level down. This in turn kept her wide awake at night, so she was given barbiturates to help her sleep." Garland herself confirms the effect of this brutal chemical regimen: "The studio became a haunted house for me." She remained a prisoner of the speed-and-downer cycle until her death in 1969—from an "incautious self-overdosage of Seconal," taken to counteract the speed she used to help her through the day.

Although the 1930s had more tabloid newspapers than today, they didn't in those days dwell on the substance abuse of celebrities. The excesses of the Hollywood studios never came to light until years later, when the old-time studio bosses like Mayer and Cohen no longer wielded power or instilled fear, and the public was at least a little more sophisticated in its reaction to drug use. The stars themselves felt more able to talk about what had been done to them, and how it amounted to nothing short of deliberate pharmaceutical child abuse. At the time, though, when Garland was turning out movies like *Pigskin Parade*, *Love Finds Andy Hardy*, and *Broadway Melody of 1938*, the public assumed the formidable zip and pep of the juvenile performer was nothing more than exuberant teen energy and good clean fun.

The great irony, however, was that the Depression-era tabloids where far from free of drug news. Harry J. Anslinger was busily demonizing marijuana, and, to a lesser extent cocaine, to consolidate the position (and budget) of his newly formed Federal Bureau of Narcotics, claiming that the demon weed would inexorably lead to mayhem, madness, and murder, and also sexual promiscuity and rape. By an odd coincidence, Benzedrine was first being marketed at approximately the same time as the Volstead Act was repealed, after a dozen years of alcohol prohibition. Anslinger had previously held office as the assistant commissioner in the Bureau of Prohibition, and much of his motivation—aside from pure megalomania, and an envy of J. Edgar Hoover and his Division of Investigation (DOI) that would change its name, in 1935, to the Federal Bureau of Investigation, the omnipotent FBI—was to provide alternative careers for prohibition agents who were out of a job when Franklin Roosevelt came to power and ended the absurd and highly corrupt ban on alcohol.

The modern temptation is to treat Anslinger as a joke, and he has even been made the subject of a campy musical, but, at the time, there was nothing funny about his propaganda campaign against "reefer madness"—fully endorsed by newspaper baron William Randolph Hearst. The Anslinger assault would shape the War on Drugs for the rest of the twentieth century, and clear on into the twenty-first, and be responsible for thousands of deaths, millions of incarcerations, trillions in criminal profits, the erosion and abuse of civil liberties, and an entire and detrimental revision of the relationship between citizens and those in authority. With Hearst's help, Anslinger attempted to create a national (and even international) drug hysteria with horror fantasies typified by this excerpt from *American Magazine*:

"An entire family was murdered by a youthful addict in Florida. When officers arrived at the home, they found the youth staggering about in a human slaughterhouse. With an axe he had killed his father, mother, two brothers, and a sister. He seemed to be in a daze… He had no recollection of having committed the multiple crimes."

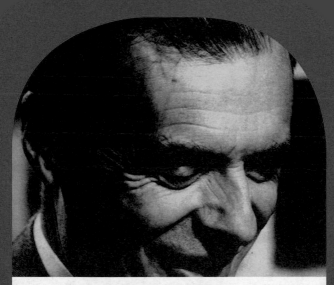

ARTIFICIAL PARADISE

AT APPROXIMATELY the same time Harry Anslinger was spreading grotesque and fabricated disinformation, Aldous Huxley summed up for the first time the basic dilemma that has, throughout the twentieth century, surrounded the very idea of recreational drugs. "That humanity at large will ever be able to dispense with Artificial Paradises seems very unlikely. Most men and women lead lives at the worst so painful, at the best so monotonous, poor, and limited that the urge to escape, the longing to transcend themselves if only for a few moments, is and has always been one of the principal appetites of the soul. Art and religion, carnivals and saturnalia, dancing and listening to oratory—all these have served, in H. G. Wells' phrase, as Doors in the Wall. And for private, for everyday use there have always been chemical intoxicants. All the vegetable sedatives and narcotics, all the euphorics that grow on trees, the hallucinogens that ripen in berries or can be squeezed from roots—all, without exception, have been known and systematically used by human beings from time immemorial. To these natural modifiers of consciousness modern science has added its quota of synthetics—chloral, for example, and Benzedrine, the bromides, and the barbiturates." ●

UNFORTUNATELY, ANSLINGER HAD A FAR LARGER, and much more gullible and ignorant congregation than Huxley, and they were more than prepared to swallow Harry J's calculated racist, anti-pot screeds like the story of "two Negros who took a girl fourteen years old and kept her for two days under the influence of hemp, and who, upon recovery, was found to be suffering from syphilis." It was also, on the surface, surprising that Anslinger concentrated with such unilateral ferocity on the innocuous cannabis, but closer examination made clear that Anslinger was more concerned with headlines and political power than the alleviation of any social menace, either real or imagined. To tell tales of multiple rape, mass murder, drugged victims, and stoned psychosis, and chase down a kid with a lid of dope, or an impoverished Mexican with a marijuana patch, was far easier that confronting any more real problem. Anslinger was being supported both politically and financially by Du-Pont, the giant chemical corporation, and it wanted him to eradicate the hemp industry, creating a competition-free market for its new man-made fibers.

Another incongruity was that Anslinger and the Federal Bureau of Narcotics showed absolutely no interest in the widespread use and abuse of Benzedrine, especially as it was beginning to demonstrate that it definitely had a darker side, especially when a habitual user was coming down off the drug. Even while Smith, Klein & French were touting Benzedrine as a manifold panacea, more independent members of the medical profession were expressing serious doubts about the protracted use of amphetamine. The textbook descriptions of a speed comedown described psychological symptoms like "insomnia, mental states resembling schizophrenia, aggressiveness, irritability, confusion, and panic." They went on to warn of how "chronic and/or extensively continuous use can lead to amphetamine psychosis, which causes delusions, depression, and paranoia." One might imagine that an agency such as the FBN might at least take an interest in a widely used chemical stimulant when doubts were starting to be expressed about the physical and social effects of its prolonged use, but Anslinger is not on record as ever having said a bad word about Benzedrine, and one can only assume he was unwilling to go up against such a powerful entity as Smith, Klein & French.

Stretching the imagination quite a bit further, the "youthful addict" who slaughtered his family, or the alleged syphilitic "negroes," had they existed at all, were more likely extreme cases of amphetamine psychosis in individuals who had been driven to madness by toking on a couple of joints. Indeed, if Anslinger had been making even a minimal attempt to run a functional federal agency to regulate drug use in the United States, he might well have investigated any possible evidence of amphetamine use by the celebrity criminals of the time, the now legendary killers and bank robbers like Bonnie Parker and Clyde Barrow, John Dillinger, or George "Baby Face" Nelson, and not allowed them to become the sole targets of his arch-rival J. Edgar Hoover and his armed G-men.

The truth about the lives and habits of all of the gangsters of the Great Depression has, of course, been seriously distorted by Hollywood myth-making and the wish fulfillments of popular culture—the real Bonnie Parker, for instance, is now inseparable from the character played by Faye Dunaway—but speculation that the violence of their headlong bank robbing, and their obvious need for notoriety and self-aggrandizement, could easily suggest that maybe their ultimately suicidal crime sprees were, at least in part, fueled by the contents of cracked-open Benzedrine inhalers.

Of all of these Dust Bowl desperadoes, "Baby Face" Nelson is by far the most likely to have been an overlooked speedfreak. Jay Robert Nash, in his highly comprehensive crime encyclopedia *Bloodletters and Badmen* describes Nelson (real name Lester Gillis) as "something out of a bad dream. Where outlaws such as 'Pretty Boy' Floyd and the Barkers would kill to protect themselves when cornered, Nelson went out of his way to murder—he loved it," and had the unique distinction of being considered too ruthless and reckless for other hardened gangsters to tolerate. Despite his boyish looks, Nelson was an unpredictable thrill-killer with an irrational and hair-trigger temper, and John Dillinger refused to rob banks with him. He had also been exiled from Chicago by no less than Al Capone as being "too violent" for Capone to control. Clearly psychopathic, Nelson had no compunction about gunning down lawmen or innocent bystanders, and ended up killing three FBI agents, more than any other criminal in history.

Obviously the suggestion that "Baby Face" Nelson's psychosis was caused, or at least exacerbated, by amphetamine is pure speculation, but it does fit what we now know of as the classic sociopath behavior pattern of the terminal speedfreak, and it should be noted that his great excesses occurred in 1934, when Benzedrine had been available for a full two years. Benzedrine was also on the market in 1933, at the time of what became known as the Kansas City Massacre, a mass slaying of four law-enforcement officers and their prisoner right outside Union Railway Station in Kansas City, Missouri. Charles Arthur "Pretty Boy" Floyd, Vernon Miller, and Adam Richetti attempted to free their running buddy, Frank Nash, from federal custody while he was being transported to the US Penitentiary at Leavenworth, Kansas, from which he had escaped. The long-term effect of the Kansas City Massacre was to tilt public opinion away from the sort of empathy shared with outlaws like Dillinger, Barrow and Parker, Floyd, and the rest. The Robin Hood mystique they had enjoyed in the hardscrabble 1930s, when banks were perceived as the villains, disappeared, and the outlaws became viewed as little more than stone killers, fit only to be hunted down and destroyed.

To postulate that maybe speed played an unrecorded part in the gangster chronicles of the 1930s may verge on the fanciful. That connection perhaps never existed in reality, but the behavioral levels of ruthless arrogance, the almost total lack of external empathy, and any sense of long-term consequences, fit all too closely to patterns that would repeat themselves over and over again as speed became increasingly integrated into multiple levels of drug-linked subculture. We will never know for sure if Bonnie and Clyde or "Baby Face" Nelson were dangerous prototype speedfreaks, but they certainly exhibited many of what became familiar symptoms.

What is certain is that the manufacturers must have been aware that the amphetamine they were marketing could, in extreme cases, lead to extreme paranoia, and in a worst-case scenario something akin to schizophrenia. Far from backing off, however, SK&F kept the inhalers and the pills not only rolling, but actually started them rolling in a whole new direction. The military had also noted the unique side effects of the failed asthma cure and became extremely interested. To the military mind, the idea of whole divisions of combat soldier, crews of warships, or airmen on bombing missions with increased stamina, and who were able to function, possibly for days on end, without either sleeping or eating was the stuff of any general's wildest and most fantastic dreams. By the end of the 1930s, the military, led by the Germans and Hitler's reconstituted Wehrmacht, were enthusiastically moving into the speed business.

"The comedown would start with flickering in the periphery of one's vision. It could resemble the flapping of tiny wings, but if you turned your eyes to look, they immediately vanished. These half-seen hallucinations may well have been what caused Hunter S. Thompson to come up with the concept of 'bat country,' a region/state-of-mind in the Nevada desert that his hero Raoul Duke drives through in the classic novel *Fear And Loathing In Las Vegas* with '...two bags of grass, seventy-five pellets of mescaline, five sheets of high-powered blotter acid, a salt shaker half full of cocaine, and a whole galaxy of multi-colored uppers, downers, screamers, laughers, and also a quart of tequila, a quart of rum, a case of Budweiser, a pint of raw ether, and two dozen amyls.' The band's disreputable Ford truck with no insurance could never boast such a cargo manifest, but we desperate rock & rollers did our level best to rise to any intoxicant occasion, which made the long drive home, clean out of everything, doubly surreal and, on occasion, triply unpleasant.

"When high, the speedfreak has a certainty of his or her own omnipotence. Sleep and hunger have been vanquished. The chimes of freedom are flashing. One talks incessantly, but hardly listens to what anyone else is saying. All things are possible except you can't remember what all things had been, 10 minutes earlier when you first enumerated them. Coming down, on the other hand was something else entirely. There was no true physical reaction as when the junkie is deprived of opiates, except maybe a jagged shaky feeling that made it hard to keep one's hands steady. The consequences were in the mind, the vision, and the perception. The drummer had the best idea. He had a habit secreting a couple of Mandrax (the British name for Quaaludes) about his person and then dropping them at the start of the journey and putting himself in a blissful coma for the whole experience. As for the rest of us, without the same medicinal forward planning, we would go home the hard way, craving a soft bed and maybe 20 milligrams (mg) of Valium.

"At first we would talk and sing, but then the interior of the vehicle would fall quiet as we retreated into our own post-high introspect. Details would crowd in, irrational irritations like the way one of the band members cleared his throat, or the shape of another's ear. The grip of paranoia would never be far away, and it would become all too easy to conjure scenarios of conspiracy and

21

betrayal, how one's jealous band mates might be plotting to get rid of you. In some ways the semi-hallucinations came as relief, the fluttering at the edge of your vision, or the grotesque imagined crowds, like Wally Wood drawings from classic 1950s issues of *Mad*, that might mysteriously gather in the fields, woods, or hedgerows beyond the hard shoulder of the highway, at least served as a reminder that nothing was as it should be, and little was really real, beyond the ceaseless driving on an endless highway in grey pre-dawn that seemed filled with unfocused specters and undefined threat." ●

SPEED FOR THE SUPER SOLDIER

IN 1938, THE BERLIN-BASED TEMMLER PHARMACEUTI-cal company began marketing a German version of meth-amphetamine under the brand name Pervitin. It rapidly became a top seller among the German civilian popula-tion, but Otto Ranke, the director of the Institute for General and Defense Physiology at Berlin's Academy of Military Medicine, had other plans. In September 1939, Ranke tested the drug on 90 university students, and not-ed the speed-dosed undergraduates clearly demonstrated increased self-confidence, concentration, and willingness to take risks, at the same time as being far less sensitive to pain, hunger and thirst, and able to go for long periods—in some cases three or four days—without sleep. Ranke be-lieved he had found the key to better-blitzkriegs-through-chemistry, and the creation of the legendary super soldier.

Once he had concluded that Pervitin could help Nazi Germany win the coming global war, Ranke was faced with the problem that time was against him. With the invasion of Poland already underway, extensive further research was clearly impossible with armies on the move, and declarations of war being made by Britain and France. Some fairly perfunctory tests were carried out on Wehrmacht military drivers during the advance into Poland, and when these confirmed the results obtained from the 90 students, Pervitin was distributed, without delay and en masse, to combat troops and air crews with hardly any restrictions. Between just April and July of 1940, more than 35 million tablets of Pervitin and Isophan (a slightly modified version produced by the Knoll pharmaceutical company) were shipped to the SS, the Wehrmacht, and the Luftwaffe in packages labeled "Stimulant," and with instructions recommending one or two 3 mg tablets should be taken "to maintain sleeplessness." Later, as though the speed itself wasn't attractive enough for the troops, it was even packaged like candy to make it super palatable. Chocolates dosed with methamphetamine were known as *Fliegerschokolade* ("flyer's chocolate") when given to pilots, or *Panzerschokolade* ("tanker's chocolate") when given to tank crews.

As the panzers rolled and the Stuka dive-bombers dropped from the sky with banshee sirens, as Hitler's seemingly unstoppable blitzkrieg stormed across Europe, swallowing Poland, France, Belgium, Holland, and large areas of Yugoslavia, the use of speed was hardly a well-kept secret. Somewhat better concealed were the increasingly clear side effects caused by the indiscriminate use of Pervitin and Isophan, and that German soldiers were drinking more heavily than might be expected, and stealing medical-kit opiates to counter the strain of the constant diet of speed. Another unfortunate fact was that the supposed super soldiers quickly developed a tolerance to the drug intended to make them super. In November of 1939, a 22-year-old soldier in occupied Poland wrote home to his family in Cologne, "It's tough out here, and I hope you'll understand if I'm only able to write to you once every two to four days soon. Today I'm writing you mainly to ask for some Pervitin." Seven months later, in May of 1940, the same soldier wrote again. "Perhaps you could get me some more Pervitin so that I can have a backup supply?" Finally, in July of the same year, another request was mailed. "If at all possible, please send me some more Pervitin." The ration of one or two 3 mg tablets didn't seem to be doing it for him. After the war, the young soldier would prove to be the writer Heinrich Böll, who in 1972 became the first German writer to be awarded the Nobel Prize for Literature after World War II.

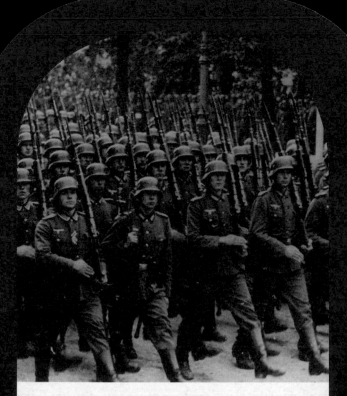

ISSUE THE DRUGS

"IN JANUARY 1942, a group of 500 German soldiers stationed on the eastern front and surrounded by the Red Army were attempting to escape. The temperature was minus 30 degrees Celsius. A military doctor assigned to the unit wrote in his report that at around midnight, six hours into their escape through snow that was waist-deep in places, 'more and more soldiers were so exhausted that they were beginning to simply lie down and freeze.' The group's commanding officers decided to give Pervitin to their troops. 'After half an hour,' the doctor wrote, 'the men began spontaneously reporting that they felt better. They began marching in orderly fashion again, their spirits improved, and they became more alert.'" ●

AS THE TIDE OF WAR TURNED AGAINST THE NAZIS, Adolf Hitler increasingly began to pin his hopes of an ultimate victory on advanced secret weapons: jet fighter planes like the Heinkel He 162, and the V1 and V2 rockets, which came to limited fruition, and were actually deployed against Southern England. The Führer was also looking to more fanciful projects, like the V10—a missile capable of hitting cities on the Eastern Seaboard of the United States—that never made it past the drawing board. The wish list for a last-ditch Nazi victory wasn't, however, confined to hardware. The Nazis final dream also included the concept of a "miracle pill" that superseded Pervitin and Isophan in chemically enhancing the performance of their troops. In March of 1944, Vice-Admiral Hellmuth Heye (who later became a member of parliament with the conservative Christian Democratic Party and head of the German parliament's defense committee) charged Kiel-based pharmacologist Gerhard Orzechowski to create a drug that would "keep soldiers ready for battle when they are asked to continue fighting beyond a period considered normal, while at the same time boosting their self-esteem."

By November 1944, Orzechowski had developed a pill that was a "cocktail" composed of 5 mg of cocaine, 3 mg of Pervitin, and 5 mg of Eukodal (a morphine-based painkiller). This new combat stimulant was code-named D-IX, and was first tested on prisoners at Sachsenhausen concentration camp. Eighteen prisoners, each carrying a 20-kilo (kg) backpack, were ordered to march continuously, and it was discovered that this group—dubbed, with grim Nazi humor, the "pill patrol"—could march without resting for up to 90 kilometers (km) a day. Although a number of the first test subjects dropped dead from the exertions, Orzechowski's records indicated that several of the forced participants in the experiment felt fine with only two or three short stops a day: "The considerable reduction of the need in sleep is very impressive. This drug disables sensations of fatigue, and increases a man's action ability and will." Essentially, D-IX turned human beings into near-robots. The results of all those tests proved so successful that plans were drawn up to supply D-IX drug to all Nazi combat troops. Fortunately, before the drug could go into mass production, the Allies had entered Germany, and the horrendous Nazi pharmaceutical dream never became reality.

MORE SCIENCE OF SPEED

THE ACTION of amphetamine in the brain causes an excess release of the chemical dopamine. This is what produces the hit, the sense of pleasure, euphoria, even omnipotence. (Dopamine is also released by exercise, chocolate, and sex, although in lesser, more controlled quantities.) Likewise, the feeling of exhaustion and depression when coming down is due to unnaturally low levels of dopamine in the brain. With heavy use, especially intravenous use, the neurons that produce dopamine may become damaged and production goes lower, and researchers are far from certain if they naturally regenerate. Even less well understood is the action of

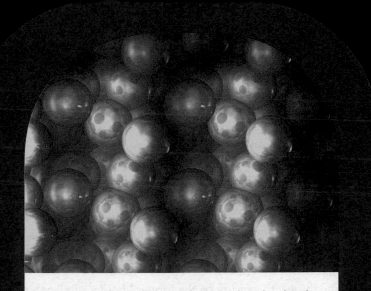

speed on serotonin levels, which are directly related to sleep. The chemical is released during the REM stage of sleep, which is disrupted by depressants and stimulants alike. It is known that serotonin is a key to growing brain tissue. (Babies dream, on average, four times as much as adults.) ●

THE GERMANS WERE NOT, HOWEVER, THE ONLY PRO-tagonists in World War II to experiment with the idea of using drugs to artificially improve the performance of their fighting men. Japan was also manufacturing its own version of Pervitin under the trade name Hiropon. The Japanese military was not as obsessive in its record-keeping as the Nazis, so it is unclear exactly how much Hiropon was distributed to the Imperial troops, but it might logically be expected to have contributed to the suicidal "no retreat, no surrender" resistance that the US Army and Marines encountered

on Iwo Jima and Okinawa, and also the kamikaze suicide attacks on allied warships.

Accounts were certainly preserved of how these kamikaze pilots were given injections of a drug called Philopon,
a liquid variation of Hiropon, before being dispatched
on the suicide missions. The kamikazes—literal transla-
tion the "divine wind"—were named for a typhoon that
had halted a seemingly unstoppable invasion of Japan in
the thirteenth century by the Mongol hordes of Genghis
Khan. Their suicide attacks on US warships were the
brainchild of Vice Admiral Takijiro Onishi, who had realized, by late 1944, Japan would be unable either to halt
the American advance across the Pacific, or to match US
industrial production at home, except by extreme and desperate measures. The kamikaze concept was simple in the
extreme. A fighter plane packed with a half-ton of explosives would be flown directly into an enemy vessel. Such a
direct hit could cripple an aircraft carrier or battleship, and
sink outright a cruiser or destroyer. Designs were actually
created for a custom-built, pilot-controlled, flying bomb,
not unlike a piloted version of the V1 rockets that the
Germans were launching at England at approximately the
same time. Unfortunately for the Japanese pilots, the US
advance was moving too quickly for these machines to go
into full production, and by far the majority of the kamikaze suicide missions were flown in aging Mitsubishi Zero
fighter planes that were too old, too long in service, and
too decrepit to ever be repaired and returned to combat.

In the West, the idea of any form of combat that
constituted a guaranteed one-way ticket to oblivion was
rarely considered as a viable strategy. Soldiers on both

sides might face seemingly hopeless odds, and near-fatal situations in which it was clear that only a small percentage would come out alive. Both Hitler and Stalin were prone to issuing grandiose orders, demanding that armies under their commands hold positions to the last man. The notion that a protracted and extensive operation in which combatants volunteered for certain death without the slightest chance of survival seems implausible and unsustainable, yet Onishi experienced no shortage of willing recruits. Thousands volunteered for the rudimentary flight training, just sufficient to enable the kamikaze pilot to get his explosive-packed plane into the air, to the target, and then dive directly into it. Most were boys in their late teens, impressionable and heavily indoctrinated, anxious to prove that their emperor and country meant more to them than their own lives. In many respects their mindset was not unlike that of modern Islamic extremists who train for suicide bombing missions, and numbers of willing kamikazes were such that they far exceeded the supply of available aircraft.

Before the kamikaze pilots took off on their terminal missions, they went through a solemn, quasi-religious, warrior ceremony, involving sake, wreaths of flowers, decorated headbands, and powerful injections of liquid amphetamine—a final act of ritual brainwashing—plus the administration of enough stimulants to keep them gung-ho crazy long enough to complete the mission.

After the Japanese surrender, a huge stockpile of Hiropon amphetamine assembled by the Japanese military was discovered, much of it already being widely distributed under the street name "shabu." With supreme irony, even though the Japanese Ministry of Health banned the traffic of speed in 1951, shabu facilitated a thriving black market in methamphetamine, controlled by organized crime families of the Yakuza in the Chiba section of Tokyo, and in other Japanese cites. To add income to irony, the speed trade in the early 1950s provided the working capital for the Yakuza to diversify its operations into everything from trucking to movie distribution. It proved to be the first time that the profits from dealing methamphetamine made possible large-scale underworld expansion, but it was far from the last.

The Allies, although supposedly the good guys of World War II, were also not above considering the use of amphetamine to enhance the performance of their troops, but at least the Allied commanders were considerably more circumspect about just how much speed was being fed to their fighting men and women. Generals like George Patton and Douglas MacArthur (and Omar Bradley, for wholly different reasons) found overt drug-peddling, even to win a war, somewhat at odds with their carefully cultivated warrior images; however, there is a wealth of anecdotal evidence suggesting that Benzedrine and Desoxyn—a more powerful version of methamphetamine first marketed by Abbott Laboratories in 1942—were widely circulated among American and British bomber crews. Give a little old lady in an English pub a couple of extra gins, and wild stories will emerge of a flourishing pill culture, especially in the months leading up to D-Day, when the British Isles were little more than a vast staging area for the invasion of Europe and also the home base of the massive Anglo/American thousand bomber raids into the heart of Germany. Many a GI or B17 tail gunner wasn't above adding a few pills to the nylons, cigarettes, and chocolate with which they wooed the local girls.

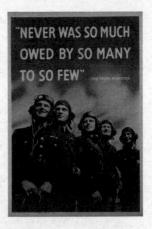

Even before the United States entered the war, when Hitler had overrun Western Europe and the British fought alone, speed was seemingly employed as a crucial combat tool. Through the summer and fall of 1940, Hermann Goering (a cross-dressing cocaine and morphine addict) and his Luftwaffe attempted to bomb London into submission, but were held at bay in the skies over Southern England by the fighter pilots of the Royal Air Force, in their Spitfires and Hurricanes, in what became known as The Battle of Britain. Vastly outnumbered by the German Messerschmidt Bf 109s that provided the fighter escort for the large, but slow-moving bomber formations, the RAF men found themselves flying two, three, and even four sorties each day. Sleep was at a premium, and the head of Fighter Command, Air Chief Marshal Sir Hugh Dowding, was supposedly advised to confront this problem by employing one of the amphetamine-based chemical stimulants already being used by his Nazi adversaries. Dowding was something of a strange individual, who, while a formidable and tireless tactician, was also a devout spiritualist who held seances to contact the spirits of the young aviators who had died under his command. At the suggestion of giving his men drugs, however, Dowding didn't balk or hesitate. According to RAF records, seemingly limitless quantities of Benzedrine tablets and inhalers were made available to his pilots.

The RAF's triumph in the Battle of Britain prompted Prime Minister Winston Churchill to make his legendary speech of national gratitude that included the lines, "British airmen who, undaunted by odds, unwearied in their constant challenge and mortal danger, are turning the tide of the World War by their prowess and by their devotion. Never in the field of human conflict was so much owed by so many to so few."

No hint was given, however, that part of the reason these heroes were "unwearied in their constant challenge" was because they had a great deal of chemical assistance.

Little evidence exists—except some unsubstantiated stories of amphetamine being the secret ingredient in GI K-rations—that speed was handed out willy-nilly to ground troops, in the manner of the Germans, but all indication are that the World War II air war—following the precedent set by Dowding during the Battle of Britain—made ample and constant use of speed, especially during the massive allied air raids on enemy cities. Issuing bennies or Desoxyn to bomber crews seems logical. Long flights over enemy occupied Europe had to be a protracted and excruciating combination of boredom, concentration, and fear, punctuated by the sudden violence of assaults by enemy fighter planes or anti-aircraft flack, culminating in the few minutes over the target when the bomb-load would be released, and then the equally lengthy and just as equally fraught flight back to home and safety. Under such prolonged and unimaginable stress, opiates or alcohol would render a crew sloppy and dysfunctional, but speed constituted the perfect stimulant in that it allowed air crews to remain sharp and efficient while at the same time it provided a psycho-chemical buffer against the drain of tension and trauma. Needless to say, the negative side of using speed inevitably manifested itself. While the American brass, for the most part, accepted a level of crew burnout and combat fatigue, the British RAF, under the command of Air Marshal Sir Arthur "Bomber" Harris—the less-than-sane architect of the firestorm obliteration of the historic city of Dresden—were somewhat Victorian in their attitudes and viewed a member of a bomber crew coming unglued as a character defect just short of cowardice, and dubbed it "Lack Of Moral Fiber." The letters "LMF" stamped on an airman's record would dog him for the rest of his career. Not all US commanders were quite as enlightened as their colleagues. As casualties mounted, tours were extended with little regard to the physical and psychological effects on their men, which created the unique form of madness so brilliantly captured in Joseph Heller's novel *Catch-22*.

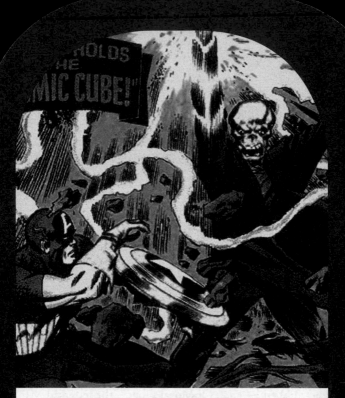

CAPTAIN AMERICA AND THE RED SKULL

THE PHARMACOLOGICAL reality of World War II was symbolically captured, and even amplified, by comic-book master Jack Kirby in the fantasy adventures of Captain America. Captain America, with his red white and blue costume and shield, starts out as a frail young man named Steve Rogers, who, despite being aware that previous test subjects had gone raving mad, volunteers to take the "Super-Soldier Serum and Vita-Ray treatment" developed by the decidedly strange Dr. Josef Reinstein. The exact formula of the serum is not specified, but it is known to be a dangerously powerful character transformer. Rogers is dosed and rayed, miraculously retains his sanity, and is transformed from the frail young man into the virtual apex of human development, with a body that is in perfect physical condition, with strength, speed, agility, dexterity, reflexes, coordination, balance, and physical endurance, and becomes Captain America, battling the Nazis and the Japanese wherever they are at their most evil and fiendish. Almost immediately he is confronted by his Nazi counterpart, the Red Skull, a grotesque figure in jackboots, green coveralls, with his head permanently encased in a grotesque and ghoulish scarlet skull mask. With his training as a super-villain and ultimate übermensch, personally supervised by no less than Adolf Hitler, and eventually also dosed with the Super-Soldier Serum, the Red Skull proves himself to be Captain America's equal but evilly opposite counterpart. Although the complex plot line of the confrontations between Captain America and the Red Skull continue to this day, and have expanded from comic books to movies, TV animation shows, and video games, Jack Kirby's inspired, fictional invention of drug-enhanced combat troops in the early 1940s still stands as a fanciful but uncomfortably accurate analogue of what was really happening. ●

ONCE THE PEACE HAD BEEN ESTABLISHED, PATTERNS of amphetamine consumption rapidly changed. In Japan, the Yakuza were pedaling shabu on the streets of Tokyo, and, in the broken-toothed, bombed out ruins of devastated Europe, Benzedrine, Pervitin and Desoxyn were only two more items on the menu in a black market, where characters like Harry Lime, in the movie classic *The Third Man*, dealt in everything from Scotch whisky, nylon stockings, and cigarettes, to antibiotics and morphine. Meanwhile, back in the United States, the leaders of a victorious, and now unbelievably wealthy nation were gearing up for the Cold War against communism, and planning the direction they believed a post-atomic civilization should follow.

Speed would play a whole and very diverse menu of roles in the post–World War II civilian world, but its military applications were by no means abandoned or forgotten. Certainly not by the Air Force, which permitted the use of amphetamines by the B-52 crews of Strategic Air Command (SAC) in 1960, and Tactical Air Command (TAC) in 1962. These were the Dr. Strangelove days of Mutually Assured Destruction (MAD), when bombers loaded with nuclear weapons flew round the clock missions to their fail-safe points and back, and it is hardly a happy thought that, even though long ago, the potential for nuclear annihilation was quite literally in the hands of airmen high on speed.

While the Air Force handed out the pills, the intelligence community maintained ongoing and evolving programs of mind-bending, mind-altering, mind-controlling pharmacology—the most notorious being the Central Intelligence Agency's (CIA) MKULTRA unit—and amphetamine would remain a major asset in the spymasters' black pharmacopoeia. When the Cold War warmed up with the escalating "police action" in Vietnam, speed was, once again, right on the front line. Even while medicine and the law were placing escalating restrictions on the prescription and use of the various brand-name amphetamines, the drug corporations maintained a strict policy of business as usual with the military. As the war in Vietnam escalated, Smith, Kline & French, Abbott Laboratories, and all the other amphetamine manufacturers were more than ready to ship unlimited quantities of their product to any firefight in the jungle. More than 225 million doses, mainly of Dexedrine, but also an amphetamine of French manufacture with the brand name Obestol were supplied to US troops during the war in Southeast Asia. The impact of that amount of stimulant to any army in the field could only have been, quite literally, mind-boggling, and adds a whole extra dimension to the popular image of the in-country US grunt as a reluctant and occasionally psychotic hero in an impossible war, smoking pot, shooting heroin, ducking for dear life, and wondering what he was doing there anyway.

To balance the increasingly obvious negative effects of an army that was being saturated with speed, most particularly an edgy, trigger-happy nervousness, loss of appetite, and insomnia, a barbiturate called Binoctal was issued in 10 and 25 mg doses, which at least allowed the grunts on the ground to sleep when otherwise it might have been impossible. At no time was any real consideration given to the long-term effects of an army that was running on a relentless cycle of uppers and downers. Only more recent studies—related to both Iraq wars—suggested that amphetamine use by troops in combat might be a definite contributory factor to PTSD (post-traumatic stress disorder).

For those among the general public who were still bothering to pay attention, it came as something of a surprise that the military was still using amphetamines as a combat stimulant as late in the day as Gulf 1 and Gulf 2. A 2004 report in the British newspaper *The Guardian* claimed that while George W. Bush was declaring from the teleprompter that "methamphetamine is a powerfully addictive drug that dramatically affects users' minds and bodies, shatters families, and threatens our communities," and that "chronic use can lead to violent behavior, paranoia, and an inability to cope with the ordinary demands of life," the Pentagon was not only distributing the drug to its men and women in the field but, in some cases, allegedly mandating they use it.

The current use of speed by the military came to light after a friendly-fire bombing incident in April 2002 near Kandahar in Afghanistan. Two US F-16 pilots, Major Harry Schmidt and Major William Umbach, mistakenly attacked a Canadian infantry unit, killing four and injuring eight. Both pilots were placed on charges, but their lawyers claimed the defendants' judgment had been impaired because they had been "pressured into taking amphetamine before the mission." The report went on to suggest that the mandatory use of speed by US fliers was common to the point of routine, service careers could be "derailed for pilots who refuse to drug themselves," and that amphetamines were also being issued to special forces, on missions which demanded they operate for more than 48 hours without sleep.

Further investigations revealed that, whatever the Americans might be using to medicate their people, the British, both in Iraq and Afghanistan, had been experimenting with a new "amphetamine-like" drug called Provigil, marketed by the Pennsylvania-based company Cephalon, and licensed in Britain to treat tiredness associated with the rare sleeping disorders narcolepsy and obstructive sleep apnea. The British Ministry of Defence denied that

Provigil or any other drug of that type had been issued to the Brit armed forces. A budget memo, however, obtained by *The Guardian* under the British "open government code" revealed that the Defence Medical Supplies Agency (DMSA)—the agency that approves and supplies medical products "to sustain UK military capability"—approved expenditures of more than $100,000 for Provigil in 2002 alone, at a time when British troops were only deployed in Afghanistan, and a year before they entered Iraq.

Meanwhile, in the private sector, drug use by employees of Blackwater Worldwide—a polite way of describing private hired-gun mercenaries working for the United States—became the subject of a 2007 inquiry after 17 civilians died in and around Nisour Square, in western Baghdad, when Blackwater guards fired into a crowd of Iraqi nationals "without provocation." According to lawyers for survivors and the families of those slain, the guards continued firing even after one of their comrades tried to stop them from shooting, and committing what the lawyers categorized as acts of "premeditated murder." Subsequent allegations claimed that at least a quarter of Blackwater security guards in Iraq use steroids and other "judgment-altering substances." No one seemed in the least surprised when one of the "judgment-altering substances"—despite a statement from Blackwater that "steroids and performance enhancement drugs, both illegal and prescribed, are absolutely in violation of our policy"—was heavily rumored to be amphetamine or some similar stimulant.

It seems inevitable that whatever the current domestic and civilian attitudes toward the use of amphetamines may be, once the shooting starts, the effects of speed, especially those of aggression and endurance, are simply too tempting to exclude from military operations.

Even the speedfreak will admit that two of the most common symptoms of prolonged amphetamine use are paranoia and obsession. Most often these traits are manifested in nothing more than an exacerbated version of common individual anxiety. People are talking about you. A specific person has a grudge against you and is plotting to do you wrong. Sexual partners are cheating on you, or business associates are robbing you or shortchanging you, cooks are spitting in your food, and the cop on the beat is eyeing you askance. In some cases, however, paranoia and obsession rise to more fancifully rarefied levels. Sometimes they are the mysteries, theories, and conspiracies that make up the popular mythology of the twentieth and twenty-first centuries—UFOs and alien abductions, the intelligence community, and the Kennedy assassinations, the hollow Earth, or how malevolent reptile men walk among us in human disguise. High on crystal meth, the self-appointed expert will lecture anyone who cares to listen (or not, as the case may be—speed-freak monologues are usually unstoppable) on the identity of the gunman on Dealey Plaza, or what really goes on inside Area 51. When not talking, the fixated speedfreak will cover legal pads or exercise books with incomprehensibly dense screeds on the subject, in cramped handwriting, complete with drawings and diagrams that cover every square inch of the page.

In more advanced cases, interminable talk may actually turn into bizarre action. Curtains will be obsessively drawn so the cops in the helicopters can't peer in. The same apartment windows will be covered in tinfoil to keep out the rays of the mind-control machine. The TV is turned off because it is talking back. The electricity in the apartment wiring has become audible. The real time to worry, of course, is when the speedfreak starts babbling about firearms and impending attack by the New World Order. At that point it is a very good idea to vacate the area.

A much more mundane form of obsession, especially among young women, is an overwhelming desire for neatness, and a need to clean up anywhere they happen to find themselves high on some variety of speed. This was and still is, needless to say, ruthlessly exploited by males of the same subculture, who, using hits of speed as lure, exploit obsessive young women as unpaid domestics. ●

SPEED FOR THE LEADER

ADOLF HITLER WAS UNRIVALED AS THE GREATEST AND, by far, the most homicidal speedfreak in history, but to acknowledge him as such is probably a mortal insult even to speedfreaks. To make any case for the Nazi regime, with its banners and uniforms, its logistically organized butchery, and micromanaged evil, was simply a result of the consumption of any drug is plainly absurd. It does, however, have to be noted that, while his armies attempted to conquer the world while swallowing Pervitin and Isophan, and were only narrowly deprived of the added boost of D-IX, their Führer, the supposed embodiment of the master race and their megalomaniac ambition, was being dosed with the most deeply weird cocktails of drugs that could be conceived and concocted by his personal physician, Dr. Theodor Morell.

For the last nine years of his life, Adolf Hitler, already a lifelong hypochondriac, violently refused—at times against the good advice of more conventional doctors like Dr. Karl Brandt, who had been attending to Hitler since 1933—to be separated from Morell. "What luck I had to meet Morell. He has saved my life." If any unfortunate pressed the point that the Morell's ministrations were perhaps less than good for the leader, Hitler was prone to fly into one of his infamous hysterical rages. A dangerous rivalry developed between Brandt and Morell, but in any argument Hitler inevitably sided with Morell, and, in response to one attempted medical intervention, he supposedly screamed, "No one has ever told me precisely what is wrong with me. Morell's method of cure is so logical that I have the greatest confidence in him. I shall follow his prescriptions to the letter."

Unfortunately, Dr. Morell's prescriptions were little short of bizarre, as detailed in the doctor's diary that was found intact after the fall of the Nazi regime, and Hitler's suicide in 1945. The injections that Morell gave Hitler multiple times a day were strange (some might says hellish) mixtures of topical cocaine, injected amphetamines, glucose, testosterone, estradiol (a steroid sex hormone and close relative of estrogen), and also corticosteroids. In addition, he was given a compound of strychnine and atropine, an extract of seminal vesicles, and numerous vitamins and "tonics." Morell did not note, though, what condition he believed he was treating with these strange concoctions.

Throughout his dark career Adolf Hitler's health was always the subject of constant observation and concern, not only on the part of the Nazi elite, but also the Allied intelligence community. Hitler was a self-proclaimed health nut, who refused to touch alcohol, a militant vegetarian with a penchant for grossing out dinner guests with detailed accounts of cattle slaughter, and a non-smoker who hated cigarettes so much that he would present an engraved gold watch to any of his inner circle who quit the habit. Additionally, Hitler was variously reputed to have suffered from irritable bowel syndrome, an irregular heartbeat, Parkinson's disease, and tertiary syphilis.

During the 1950s, a slew of memoirs were published by valets, photographers, chauffeurs, and other rank and file individuals who worked on the fringes of Hitler's inner circle. All describe Hitler as an increasingly sick man. His rages and mood swings were famous, but he also showed signs of gastrointestinal symptoms, skin lesions, and the kind of muscular tremors associated with Parkinson's. A similar picture is painted in the book *Inside the Third Reich* by Albert Speer, Hitler's chief architect and later his Minister for Armaments, who wrote his highly revealing—if also self-justifying—memoirs after serving 20 years in jail for war crimes, and participation in slave-labor projects.

Speer, who was far closer to Hitler than any of the hired help, saw just how important Morell's ever-ready needles were to the Nazi leader. Hitler, who rarely rose from his bed before noon, could, at the start of the day, be close to paralyzed by depression until Morell's first injection—what a junkie would call an eye opener. Within minutes Hitler would undergo a diametric mood swing close to a full personality change. He was suddenly animated, motivated, and highly talkative. He would claim divine inspiration and a "direct line to God." He would

47

fix on a topic or a grand design, and become wholly obsessive about it, but then, after maybe four or five hours,
according to the circumstance, he would start to flag, his
attention would wander, and he'd become more prone to
either irrational rages or bouts of convoluted paranoia. If
only for the protection of those around him, Morell would
be summoned with his hypodermic, and the reanimated
leader would repeat the cycle, often deep into the night as
long as Morell kept giving him the shots.

Although Morell managed to insinuate himself with
Propaganda Minister Joseph Goebbels and his family,
many of the Nazi elite loathed the always-on-call Morell.
Goering, one of the very few among the Nazi leadership
who was not afraid of Hitler, openly nicknamed Morell
"*Der Reichsspritzenmeister*", variously translated as "Reich Injection Master" or the "The Master of the Imperial
Needle." Even the airheaded Eva Braun, Hitler's longtime
mistress, and his wife for the last few hours of their lives,
had at first submitted herself to shots from the Injection
Master, but then turned against Morell, calling him a
"pig," and his surgery and consulting room, that sounded,
in some accounts, not unlike an alchemist's layer, "the pig
sty." Braun refused to have any more dealings with Morell,
preferring instead to drink champagne and perhaps pop
some of the ever abundant Pervitin

This dislike of Morell by the top hierarchy of the
Third Reich, however, did not stop the eccentric doctor
from accompanying Hitler on many historic excursions
both before and during World War II. In 1939 Morell,
for example, was at Hitler's side during the meetings that
led to the forced annexation of Czechoslovakia. When the

Czechoslovakian president, Emil Hacha, attempted to negotiate with Hitler instead of simply capitulating, Hitler flew into a rage, so terrifying Hacha that he fainted. Morell was immediately called to administer an injection to revive Hacha. Morell later claimed the shot was nothing more than vitamins, but the general opinion was that it was actually methamphetamine, plus the usual dubious additives. Once conscious again, the now very shaky Czech president immediately caved in to all of Hitler's demands.

A few anecdotal accounts claim that, long before Morell was shooting up Hitler with speed cocktails on a daily basis, the Führer was no stranger to speed. Stories have circulated that, prior to addressing the huge Nazi rallies—the kind depicted in the Leni Riefenstahl film *Triumph of the Will*, with banners, flaming torches, and sinister, almost Busby Berkeley choreography—Hitler would take speed, perhaps imported Benzedrine, or later Pervitin, to raise his energy levels as a performer, and counter it with a downer like phenobarbital to take the edge off the jitters and allow him more control. In this, Hitler was in total contrast to his rival, Winston Churchill, the other great orator of the World War II, who would down multiple shots of cognac before his now legendary speeches.

Whether or not Hitler's romance with amphetamine started with Morell, the detrimental effects were increasingly visible, both in his appearance and behavior, especially towards the end of his regime, when he became irrationally more ready to embrace grandiose, but highly delusional concepts, while high as a swastika-decorated kite. Film shot of Hitler between the failed July 1944 bomb plot at Hitler's Wolfsschanze ("Wolf's Lair")

Headquarters, at Rastenburg, in which Hitler narrowly escaped death, and his suicide in April 1945—including the famous and often shown last footage of him handing out Iron Crosses and chocolate eclairs to the 11- and 12-year-old Hitler Youths who were pointlessly defending Berlin against Russians—show a figure in total decay. In another fragment of film from those final days, Hitler deliberately hides his left hand behind his back to conceal an uncontrollable trembling. While Hitler's inner circle said nothing and pretended the Führer was in robust good health, British, US and Russian intelligence services all entertained the possibility that Hitler had Parkinson's, but were unaware of the vast doses of speed, coke, and steroids, plus all the other more voodoo compounds being administered by Dr. Morell.

It is, of course, quite possible that Hitler's degeneration was a result of Parkinson's or some other natural medical condition, but this would seem to be made less likely by the accounts of the final days in his underground Berlin bunker, during which, for long periods of the day, provided Morell was close at hand, Hitler, exhibited no Parkinson's symptoms or impaired speech. Quite the reverse was true. The Führer behaved with a semblance of distorted rationality, planning complex strategic and tactical moves to drive the Russians back from Berlin, and prevent the Red Army from encircling the German capital. The only problem was that the wooden pointers that he was so animatedly moving around the map table represented armies that had already been wholly wiped out, and his divorce from reality was so close to total that, when the anyone dared to give the leader an accurate appraisal of how desperate the battle for Berlin had become, Hitler refused to acknowledge the truth. General observation of speedfreaks, especially the extreme victims of the methamphetamine plague of the last 15 years, shows Hitler conforming to very similar mental and physical symptoms that can be seen in today's terminal crystal meth addicts. In all fairness, though, no meth tweaker ever set in motion the deliberate slaughter of tens of millions of human beings—except maybe in their dreams.

Although it cannot be proved beyond all reasonable doubt. The sporting odds and the safe assumption are that the meth, the cocaine, and all the outright poisons pumped into Adolf Hitler by Dr. Theodor Morell, were the cause of his bodily decay and mental detachment. Hitler, however, was not the only world leader to use amphetamine as the fuel of his rule.

ƧIR AMPHETAMINE

ONE OF the most elevated examples of how amphetamine may not be the most ideal medication for a head of state was no less than the British Prime Minister, Sir Anthony Eden. Before reaching the premiership, the suave, good-looking, debonair Eden had been a close-to-brilliant Foreign Secretary all through World War II and for 10 years of the Cold War. When, however, he succeeded Winston Churchill as prime minister in 1955, he seemed— putting it bluntly— to lose his mind. His ability to make decisions seemed to desert him, and the culmination of this less- than-rational behavior came

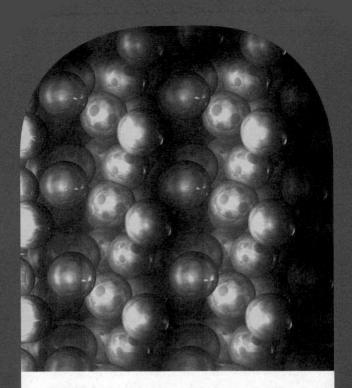

in 1956, when Sir Anthony took totally illogical military action against Egypt over the Suez Canal. His mistake in dispatching British troops to Suez is among the most enduring mysteries of modern politics. Rumors have circulated for decades that Eden, who was Prime Minister from 1955 to 1957, and was suffering from a debilitating illness at the height of the 1956 crisis, may have been taking addictive, painkilling drugs that could have clouded his judgment. Private papers recently uncovered in the Eden family archives provide a definitive answer. Eden had become a speedfreak and was being regularly prescribed a powerful combination of amphetamines and barbiturates called Drinamyl. Better known in postwar Britain as "purple hearts," they already had a reputation for impairing judgment, causing paranoia and even making the user lose contact with reality. Indeed, some years later, when The Who recorded their hit "My Generation," Roger Daltrey's stammering vocal is a deliberate parody of a mod after too many Drinamyl, a condition called "blocked" by pillheads on the street. ●

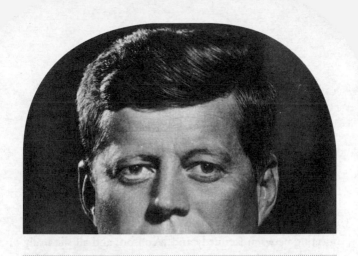

THE KENNEDY MEDICATION

WITH A CHRONICALLY DAMAGED SPINE AND ADDI-son's disease, a rare endocrine disorder, that, during and even before his presidency was a closely guarded and heav-ily concealed secret, John F. Kennedy constantly searched for better and more efficient painkillers. He could only have figured he'd found the panacea of his dreams when he ran into Dr. Max Jacobson, the original 1960s "Dr. Feel-good," who, at the time, was servicing the New York jet set—from Tennessee Williams to Bob Fosse, plus count-less drag queens and fashion models—with shots of me-thedrine and B12. How JFK and Max Jacobson first en-countered each other is less than clear, but it would seem likely that it occurred at some New York upper-crust party in the late 1950s, when Kennedy was still a Senator. Ja-cobson cruised the periphery of the Manhattan smart set, partly for the pure pleasure of hobnobbing with the rich and chic, but also trolling for new patients/customers.

Brigid Berlin (also known as Brigit Polk when she be-came an Andy Warhol "superstar") was a child of New York society and Swiss finishing schools who was sent by her mother—a close friend of Lyndon Johnson's and J. Edgar Hoover's—to the family doctor at the age of 11 to get amphetamines and Dexedrine (little orange hearts) to control her weight. In an act of rebellion, she became a formidable speedfreak and attached herself to the Warhol Factory. Berlin probably comes closest to any actual recall of the earliest meeting between Kennedy and Jacobson, and all she really remembers is that "Everyone was doing it. Jack and Jackie Kennedy definitely went to Max Jacobson's."

Jack Kennedy, however, went further than just going to Max Jacobson's. The relationship between New York's Dr. Feelgood and Kennedy became uncomfortably close to the one between Adolf Hitler and Theodor Morell. Jacobson was with Kennedy through JFK's successful victory over Richard Nixon, and then he became a regular feature at the White House. He accompanied Kennedy as part of the presidential entourage to the Vienna summit in 1961 with Nikita Khrushchev, throughout which Kennedy was sick and seriously weakened by Addison's disease, and Jacobson administered amphetamines at regular intervals both to treat and conceal Kennedy's extreme fatigue. The combination of Kennedy's ill health and Jacobson's shots may actually have had a profound, if not disastrous effect on US-Soviet relations, and future foreign policy.

At one televised session with the Russian leader, Kennedy's strength gave out, and he floundered seriously. The world saw JFK totally unable to make a convincing case for free-market capitalism in the face of a robust Khrushchev diatribe on the superiority of Marxism, complete with the coarse peasant humor that was the hallmark of Khrushchev's public persona. The meeting left Khrushchev with the distinct impression that this new, young US president was a weakling who could be easily pushed around. Based on this uninspiring first impression, Khrushchev began to operate with a heightened belligerence, leaning on Kennedy by cutting Berlin in two with a wall, and placing Soviet missiles in Cuba.

Back in Washington, Dr. Max began to conjure more exotic treatments and started injecting Kennedy, almost daily, with speedballs of vitamins, animal placentas and methedrine. Meanwhile, Kennedy's more conventional medical advisors—mostly unaware of the weirdness that Max Jacobson was pumping into the president's buttocks —were treating him with the steroid cortisone. Before press conferences and televised speeches, Kennedy's doctors increased his cortisone dose to help him handle the associated stress, and there must have been moments when Jack Kennedy felt he was going in all directions at once. Singer Eddie Fisher, who was also a devoted client/patient of Dr. Max, recalled in his biography, *Eddie: My Life, My Loves*, "Looking back on it, it's amazing how we all just accepted the fact that the president was taking Dr. Feelgood with him to meetings that would affect the entire world. The fate of the free world rested on Max's injections. I can still see Dr. Max taking a little from this bottle, a little from that one, and pull down your pants, Mr. President."

During the Cuban Missile Crisis of 1962, as Kennedy and Nikita Khrushchev faced each other across the nuclear abyss, the president was mixing mood-modulating steroids and amphetamines, along with Demerol, Methadone, Ritalin, Librium, plus miscellaneous barbiturates. A 1972 *New York Times* report quotes a doctor treating Kennedy who allegedly warned him about amphetamine use and the influence of Max Jacobson. "No president with his finger on the red button has any business taking stuff like that." Between Jack Kennedy and his brother Bobby on one side, and Nikita Khrushchev and his Kremlin advisors on the other, a tricky and tortuous course was steered with ingenious dexterous around a global nuclear holocaust. Whether the world was saved by a streak of blind luck, or the drugs JFK was taking, for once, provided a form of positive support during the twentieth century's most planet-threatening crisis can only be a matter of deep conjecture, but we did survive.

In the case of Hitler, we saw the man through to the end, and the disastrous physical and mental effects at least in part created by the amphetamines fed to him by Theodor Morell. Jack Kennedy was, of course, assassinated in Dallas, Texas. (Either by lone gunman Lee Oswald, or an elaborate coup d'état involving the Mob and the CIA—you choose.) He didn't live long enough for the world to see what Max Jacobson and his speed might have done to him in the long term.

....

THE PSYCHO-CIVILIZED SOCIETY

NOT WITHOUT A CERTAIN IRONY, JACK KENNEDY'S use of speed constituted a swan song for the drug in the conventional and chemically conservative world. Throughout the 1950s, amphetamine had been viewed as a possible factor in what some saw as the perfect post–World

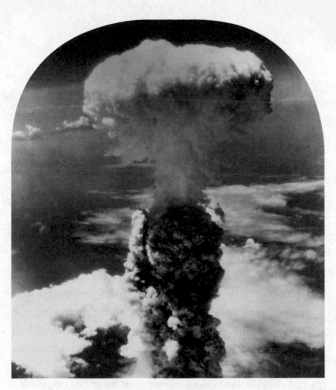

War II social order. The United States had entered World War II still reeling from the Great Depression, but by the end of the conflict, it was not only the planet's wealthiest superpower, it also had perfected an atomic weapon. The United States assumed, for a short while, that it would be able to enforce a worldwide "pax Americana," until the Soviet Union tested a nuke of its own. Large parts of Europe were devastated; the British Empire was fragmented as colonial nations demanded independence; the Soviet Union mourned more than 12 million dead; a number of Japanese cities were in ruins, and Hiroshima and Nagasaki were radioactive. In many respects, the peace presented almost as much of a challenge as the war.

In addition to its newly acquired economic, military, and nuclear power, the United States had the great advantage that no fighting had taken place on North American soil, and American cities had never been subjected to a single air raid. Its homeland infrastructure was wholly intact; US industrial capacity, that had experienced quantum growth through the war years, was unequalled, and that was all new. From breadlines, the New Deal, and a struggle for economic survival, America had moved to the point where it could do just about anything. From sea to shining sea, the nation was a blank slate on which any Utopian concept could be written. The only fly in the postwar ointment was that the United States had a new enemy. Nazi Germany may have been defeated, but the Soviet Union had overrun all of Eastern Europe and half of Germany, and was relentlessly imposing a communist system and ideology on what amounted to its newly acquired empire. That was nothing short of an anathema to those in power in the United States. As always, the majority of the US ruling elite came from the single percentile that owned 90 percent of the wealth, and had the most to lose should that wealth ever be redistributed under some form of socialism.

The fear of losing what they had, especially after the Soviets tested their first nuclear weapon, produced an almost Newtonian social pressure for capitalism to be both equal and opposite to everything communism had to offer. That pressure supplied and shaped the momentum for an American vision of the second half of the twentieth century that was one of such rigid and uniform consumer conformity that, in hindsight, was more totalitarian that Utopian. If a single location had to be chosen as the material symbol of the new America of power and abundance, Levittown, New York would have been close to the top of any list. Levittown was a subdivision on Long Island that would become the archetype of the planned postwar community. It was the first truly mass-produced suburb, and was reproduced with minor local variations throughout the country during the late 1940s and early 1950s. The brave new world being designed for the victors of World War II seemed to be one of blue collar production line workers performing constantly repetitive tasks, or white collar, grey flannel suits carrying their briefcases to nebulous jobs in the city, all traveling on the same commuter train, or driving the same freeway. Typists would tap out endless letters in the vast typing pools of pre-computer offices, while homemakers would cook, dust, and vacuum, waiting dutifully for their spouses to return.

How men who had fought their way across Europe, or the islands of the Pacific, or women who had worked in aircraft or munitions factories while the men were away, could settle to this quasi-Stepford, sanitized, hive-like existence remains a lasting mystery. One part of the answer may just possibly have been the drugs being aggressively marketed to them in the years immediately after World War II, along with all the automobiles, appliances, TV sets, breakfast cereals, cigarettes, and the rest of the panoply of consumer products being promoted as the measure of success in this transformed nation so bent on uniformity. The truth was that, for all their gaudy packaging and seeming variety, the shelves of the newly invented supermarkets really offered very little choice beyond gimmicky variations between competing brand names, and actually constituted a form of regimentation that left very little room for individualism and (heaven forbid) any form of iconoclasm.

Even some quasi-iconoclasts of the time became participants in the speed fad. Hugh Hefner, publisher of the
then-risque magazine *Playboy*, not only had his trademark
pipe and pajamas, his high-tech circular bed, his endless
parade of bikini babes, but he also, according to legend,
maintained an ample supply of Dexedrine.

One could conceivably weave an elaborate conspiracy
theory around the unilateral consumerism of the mid-
twentieth century. Fantasies could be conjured of shadowy
cabals, with representatives of the government, the military
industrial complex, the oil barons, and heads of all the manufacturing industries, including pharmaceuticals, gathering
in super secret conference to design and structure a world of
peace and prosperity in which boundaries were so absolute
that any deviation was close to impossible.

While the entertainment industry offered *Leave It to
Beaver*, *Father Knows Best*, *Ozzie and Harriet*, *I Love Lucy*,
Rawhide, and *Dragnet* as morality vignettes, the pharmaceutical giants, the tobacco manufacturers, and the liquor
industry, contributed what would amount to a four-way
balancing act of stimulants and intoxicants of nicotine,
alcohol, pep pills, and tranquilizers. As the new suburbs
grew, connected by a growing network of six-lane super-
highways, the inhabitants would be working and playing
to the synaptic drumbeat of measured chemical cocktails
in which speed would be the primary motivator, until put
to rest by a couple of martinis and bring-'em-down doses
of barbiturates, or early tranquilizers like Miltowns. The
speed in the equation was packaged as everything from
anti-depressants to diet aids. Yellow Dexedrine pills, and
black Durophet capsules put the workforce and the home-

makers into teeth-grinding action, while the slightly more problematic Drinamyl took the edge off the rush by combining amphetamine and barbiturate in one pill.

Maybe such a conspiracy theory verges on the fantastic, and the conformity of the 1950s and early 1960s evolved from nothing more than single-minded consumer osmosis. The goal was merely that of the perfect capitalist culture, and commerce acted accordingly, all with the same interests, and all moving inevitably in the same direction, but without any shadowy master-plan, or secret meetings of the power elite. Oddly, though, a recurrent phrase crops up with sufficient regularity, especially in the history of the highly active Cold War intelligence community. The phrase is "the psycho-civilized society."

MKULTRA

THE IDENTITY of whoever first coined the term "psycho-civilized society" has unfortunately been consigned to the shredder of history, but the Vegas odds are that he held a high-level position at the Central Intelligence Agency, probably from its very inception in 1947. From the start, the CIA, along with other sections of the US intelligence community, had always been extremely interested in mind-altering drugs. Via clandestine endeavors like Operation Paperclip, the CIA had inherited teams of Nazi scientists and entire libraries of meticulous Nazi records, including some of the truly demonic medical tests carried out on prisoners at Dachau and Auschwitz. By the 1950s, the bulk of secret CIA research into drugs and mind control had coalesced into the department known, at the time to only a select few, as MKULTRA, and headed by the decidedly bizarre Dr. Sidney Gottlieb. Initially the concentration was on the use of LSD and methamphetamine as tools of interrogation, and as stimulants and PsyOps tools by agents in the field. One fictional reference to this occurs in the Ian Fleming novel *Live and Let Die*. Speed is included in James Bond's briefcase of tricks, and Bond later credits the pills with preventing him from fainting after severe injury. In another Bond adventure, *Casino Royale*, the evil Le Chiffre habitually inhales Benzedrine. As Gottlieb's vision of MKULTRA broadened and became more grandiose, he and his superiors, all the way up to Director of Central Intelligence Allen Dulles, began to consider the use of drugs to control mass behavior, and even to standardize the thinking of entire populations. ●

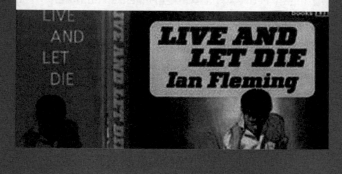

ONCE MORE THOUGH, IT WOULD BE THE DETRImental effect of protracted amphetamine use that would derail the consumer drug culture of the period. For Gottlieb, Dulles and others of their kind, a world of chemical control and conformity seemed right around the corner, but these advocates of a controlled workers' paradise had conveniently ignored a fatal flaw. As we have already seen, speed is always a double-edged sword. The heavily promoted stay-at-home homemaker was among the first to show the negative effects. They had been conditioned into accepting as their tasks cooking and dusting, vacuuming and doing laundry, organizing bridge parties or taking lessons in flower arranging, then in the night dark of the bedroom, fucking their breadwinner husbands with dutiful enthusiasm. That was the cultural propaganda carried by every medium from soap operas, to TV advertising, to *Good Housekeeping* magazine, except, of course for the part about sex. That was never mentioned, except by Alfred Kinsey in his 1953 best seller *Sexual Behavior in the Human Female* that, at the time, scandalized the nation with its insight into the reality of what was really happening in those Levittown bedrooms and elsewhere.

That suburban anthill idyll, though, after a number of years of trying to live up to the models presented by the media, was compromised by the home-making amphetamine consumers complaining of what was euphemistically categorized as "nerves" or in extreme cases "nervous collapse." The syndrome was later celebrated in two rock & roll songs—The Rolling Stones' "Mother's Little Helper," in which relief from domestic stress is found in "a little yellow pill," and Shel Silverstein's "The Ballad of Lucy Jordan," made famous by Marianne Faithfull, in which, driven insane by suburban boredom, and the knowledge that she'd "never ride through Paris in a sports car with the warm wind in her hair," housewife Lucy Jordan climbs up on the roof of the house with a "white suburban bedroom in a white suburban town" when "all the laughter grew too loud," and waits until she's led "down to the long white car that waited past the crowd."

As the 1950s drew to a close, even those in power could hear the same laughter growing louder in a culture that was obviously on a direct course to becoming pill happy. By 1958, amphetamine pills were being manufactured by the billions, but a year later, America took a step back from excessive use of the drug. 1959 saw the over-the-counter Benzedrine inhalers taken off the market, and by 1965 any product containing amphetamine became available by prescription only. Doctors were pressured by the FDA to be much more circumspect about how and to which of their patients they prescribed it, although enough corrupt "croakers" were handy enough with their pens to maintain a healthy black market in pills, and if the doctors refused to write sufficient scripts for the demand, then, hey, a new source of profit was offered to thieves willing to break into drug stores, or knock over pharmaceutical warehouses. As the importation or possession of non-prescribed amphetamines became illegal, the whole speed business became an outlaw enterprise, and the drug began to be increasingly associated with the beatnik, the bohemian, the biker, and the gay underground.

Even the mind control visions of the CIA's MKUL-TRA were turning to the possibilities of another drug—lysergic acid diethylamide, also known as LSD-25, LSD, or simply acid. Bizarre experiments were conducted on soldiers, and federal prisoners, some of whom were reputedly subjected to massive doses for extended periods of time, and driven partially insane in the process. Strangest of all was the work of CIA field agent Charles White, who was paying San Francisco prostitutes to spike their unsuspecting johns with acid, as agency operatives filmed the resulting freak-outs from behind one-way mirrors. ●

MOTHER'S LITTLE HELPER

ONE WOMAN who had developed a taste for amphetamine-based "diet pills" of the 1950s, and certainly didn't want them taken away by any government mandate, was a Memphis housewife called Gladys Presley. She lived in near-poverty, in low-income housing, with a shiftless and frequently unemployed husband, and a dangerously handsome son who played guitar and earned enough from driving a truck for an electrical contractor to buy his clothes at the store called Lansky's on Beale Street, where the city's pimps acquired their raiment. The legend has always been that Elvis Presley was introduced to speed by his platoon sergeant, while a draftee in the US Army, to keep him awake during night maneuvers in Germany. Opposing tales, however, claim that even before fame and fortune fell on him, Elvis would steal his mother's diet pills, not only to use himself, but also as a means of ensuring his popularity among the other wannabe rockabillies in and around Memphis. Before cutting his first record for Sam Phillips at Sun Records, the young Presley seemingly had a reputation for dressing "colored," and always having a supply of uppers. After his first recording had been released, and Elvis was touring almost without a break, his pill use

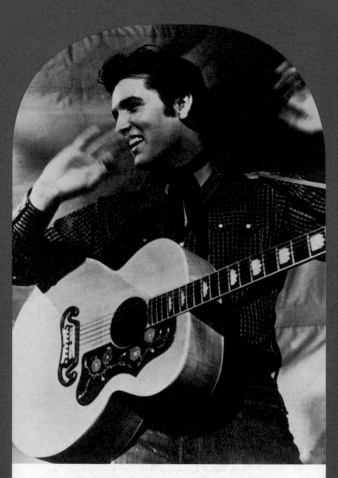

simply escalated. Guitarist Scotty Moore has told how the young Elvis was so hyper after a show that Moore and bass player Bill Black would have to walk him around for hours simply to calm him down. The foundations were clearly being laid for the paradoxical situation in which Elvis Presley would be become both a global icon, and also wholly synonymous with world-class prescription drug abuse. ●

METHEDRINE MELODIES

THE ACCOUNTS OF ELVIS STEALING HIS MOM'S DIET pills were oddly symbolic of speed's new role in society. Having proved itself incapable of creating an always-busy lockstep conformity, amphetamine's next home was among the artists of the demimonde. Jack Kerouac had, according to myth, already written *On The Road* in 20 days, whacked out of his head on Benzedrine and coffee, creating the legendary confessional scroll—the paper role from an accounting machine that saved him having to insert fresh paper into the typewriter. The suggestion has also been made that Jackson Pollock's technique of flinging, dripping, pouring, and spattering paint, as the painter energetically moved around a horizontal canvas, as though dancing, was also fueled by Benzedrine. Philip K. Dick, considered by many to be both the founder and master of modern science fiction, created his classic works *Do Androids Dream Of Electric Sheep?*, later adapted as the movie *Blade Runner*, and *Through A Scanner Darkly* in the grip of a fantastic, amphetamine-induced mind-tweak.

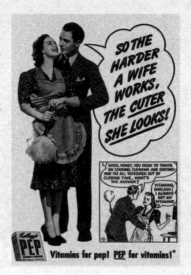

The early-to-mid-1960s saw the "Dr. Max" era in fashionable Manhattan, when Max Jacobson was injecting just about every Broadway dancer and successful fashion model with cocktails of methedrine and vitamin B12. Choreographer and film director Bob Fosse swallowed Dexedrine on a daily—sometime hourly—basis to maintain his obsessive and perfectionist work schedule, and Tennessee Williams used it to rouse himself to write from stupor of booze and barbiturates. The art-poet, anti-band The Fugs even parodied the speed vogue of the early sixties with their song *New Amphetamine Shriek:*

> *I don't have a bedtime, I don't have to come,*
> *Since I became an amphetamine bum.*

This was also the time when the Andy Warhol Factory, with its attendant freaks, velvets, and self-proclaimed superstars, was never short of either uppers or barbiturates.

Some like former socialite, former model, and supposed paramour of Bob Dylan, Edie Sedgwick, favored the latter. They, taken in tandem with booze, would ultimately kill her at the age of twenty eight. Other Warhol superstars like Holly Woodlawn and Jackie Curtis went in totally the opposite direction, and at high velocity. They were speed-freaks all the way. Warhol transvestite superstar Holly Woodlawn recalls those times in her autobiography *A Low Life in High Heels*. "Methedrine, melba toast, and a strong cup of coffee were always the eye opener, and got me ready for the rigorous task of dressing for the night ahead. There were always occasions when (Jackie) Curtis had shot too much speed and came out looking like a Picasso with one eye on her cheek and the other on her forehead."

Another Warhol superstar Ultra Violet, in her autobiography *Famous For 15 Minutes: My Years with Andy Warhol*, describes the 1966 scene at one of the Warhol live productions—The Exploding Plastic Inevitable—that were staged at the Dom on St. Mark's Place in Manhattan's East Village. The Velvet Underground were the house band and featured attraction, and Gerard Malanga also performed his notorious sadomasochistic whip dance for a very mixed audience of "art people, society people, film people, drag queens, druggies, voyeurs, tourists, rock freaks, and kids, kids, kids. Andy and I watched the whole scene from the balcony. The sound of the whip cracking on someone's back is amplified with a mike; so is the stomping of black leather boots, and the rattling of chains to the rhythm of drums and tambourines. To add to the vision of hell, strobe lights, the first in town, assault your sight, making you blink eighty times in thirty seconds. Ondine, the Queen of Drugs, and

CHAPTER FOUR

Brigid (Berlin), the Duchess, patrol the crowd and shoot up anyone who offers a hip or an arm. There's a choice of amphetamine, acid, homemade speed, Methedrine, Obetrol, Desoxyn, heroin, and Placidyl. Desoxyn is the most expensive. Drug addicts in a hurry get poked right through their pants or jeans. It takes someone with a good technique to be able to shoot through jeans, (and) Ondine's hand has a tendency to shake, but practice makes perfect. One time, Ondine punctures an artery, and his jetting blood hits a light, projecting gore onto the screen. The kids love it. Life was cheap in the sixties, as it always is in time of war, whether Vietnam or the Drug Holocaust."

At approximately the same time, on the other side of the Atlantic, different, if somewhat related, scenes were being staged that demonstrated the closeness of amphetamine to the core of the British mod movement in the mid 1960s. This could easily be observed during the months in early 1966 when The Who—boasting they performed "maximum R&B"—played an extended Tuesday night residency at London's then fashionable Marquee Club. The line outside the club would start to form in the late afternoon, and one individual who is now a well respected English music business entrepreneur, sold pills to those driven fans, the majority being obsessive and flashily dressed young men, who showed up early to guarantee they not only made it into the club before the "House Full" sign went up, but also, if possible secured a vantage point close to the stage.

The pills, nicknamed "purple hearts," "French blues," and "SKF dexies" initiated a gradually building, but nonetheless frenetic anticipation for a band that would climax their show, as high as any of the swaying, teeth-grinding audience, with Pete Townshend, swinging his right arm like a human windmill, creating ear-bleeding feedback, Keith Moon pounding a double drum kit, sometimes literally to matchwood, Roger Daltrey swinging a microphone danger-ously close to the bobbing heads of the massed mods, while John Entwistle's bass maintained a rock-solid fulcrum so the others' violent chaos could move the crowd to a glorious mass psychosis. At the very peak as Townshend rammed his already crippled guitar into a wall of speakers, the whole environment threatened to explode. For any mod warned of the long-term dangers of handful upon handful of pills, The Who had the perfect comeback: "*I hope I die before I get old.*" In a contemporary interview with Barry Miles for the un-derground newspaper *IT*, Townshend confirmed the auto-destructive, speed-driven rage of The Who. "Some nights I feel like strapping dynamite round my head and blowing up myself, the band, and the whole place."

Seemingly, by its very nature, the rock & roll of the 1960s and 1970s totally adopted speed as its primary drug of choice. Speed had never been a jazz drug. Legendary dope-users like Miles Davis would, as Miles admits in his autobi-ography, do just about anything for cocaine, but speed was far beneath Davis' well honed be-bop cool contempt. As far as Miles was concerned, speed was for ignorant crackers. As far as the music world was concerned, that was pretty much the drug's history. Country music bands, traveling hundreds of highway and back-road miles on rickety buses with their shitkicker names painted on the side, bought white crosses and black beauties, and maybe even a jar of moonshine from the same hick-town lowlifes who supplied the truck-ers, the hot-rodders and the local motorcycle hoods at the very same truck stops. Speed legends are a recurrent thread in the embroidered cowboy shirt of country and western history. The iconic images are vivid; Hank Williams dead at age 29, in the back of the Coupe de Ville, worn out by booze, speed, and morphine, surrounded by beer cans and the hand-written lyrics to an unrecorded song, "Then Came That Fateful Day."

Or Johnny Cash finding himself busted at El Paso airport with 668 Dexedrine, 475 Equanil, and thousands of dollars in cash stuffed in his pockets and inside a guitar. By his own account the country star was firmly in the grip of fear and loathing. He recreated this inner speed-turmoil in his 1975 autobiography, *The Man In Black*. "I'd talk to the demons and they'd talk right back to me—and I could *hear* them. I mean they'd say, 'Go on John, take 20 more milligrams of Dexedrine, you'll be all right.'" The Man in Black had just flown in from Ciudad Juarez, the Mexican town just across the Rio Grande from El Paso, and well known to speedfreaks in the south as an easy place to score. In this instance, after Cash had pleaded exhaustion, after months of one-night stands had brought him to the point of ceasing to care about either his actions or their consequences. "I would like to ask for leniency from the court. I know I have made a terrible mistake and would like to go back to rebuilding the image I had before this happened. The judge seemingly bought the story and gave Cash a celebrity break. He was let off with a $1,000 fine and a 30-day suspended jail sentence, to which Cash responded with the single word, "Hallelujah."

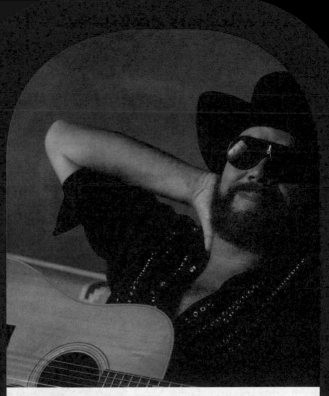

HANK DID IT THIʃ WAY

HANK WILLIAMS JR., son of the legendary singer and songwriter, described in a radio interview just how seductive pills—as opposed to alcohol—could be for country musicians on the road. "Fifteen minutes after taking a few pills the whole world took on a rosy glow and pretty soon I started to see what Daddy and Johnny Cash saw in the stuff. With liquor you'd always have to face the inevitable morning after with your mouth feeling like used steel wool and your temples trying to figure out a way to get out of your head. With pills you can postpone that morning after for a hell of a long time, weeks in fact and also you could play the shows all night if you wanted to." ●

IN THE HILLBILLY SOUTH, THE FIRST IMPACT OF rock & roll was little more than a quickening of tempo and new names on the sides of the buses. Instead of Bob Wills and the Texas Playboys, the truck stops began to see Elvis Presley and the Blue Moon Boys, Buddy Holly and the Crickets, Gene Vincent and the Bluecaps, but the old ways of honky-tonking, and patterns of drug and booze consumption would remain relatively unchanged. Two decades after Hank Williams' death, rock pioneer Gene Vincent would die in uncomfortably

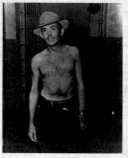

HANK WILLIAMS

similar circumstances at an uncomfortably similar age. In Europe—especially England—the same menu of amphetamine pills was playing virtually the same central role, except it came from a slightly different source.

The Beatles learned the value of being able to stay awake for days on end—and also the sexual advantages of speed—in Germany during their house-bands stints among the strippers, whores, and whip-wielding dominatrices on Hamburg's notorious Reeperbahn. Nowhere, though, was amphetamine more readily embraced than by the mods of London in the early 1960s. Unlike in the United States, where speed had a rural and small town reputation, English uppers were the urban/suburban drug. It was used by factory workers to cure their hangovers after a rough night at the pub. It was what the girls in the typing pool used to lose weight, and distance themselves from the mind-numbing keyboard. Among the young, it made possible non-stop *Clockwork Orange* weekends of rowdyism, night-clubbing, obsessive dancing, and, on occasion, outbreaks of mindless violence, which would culminate, on long holiday weekends, in pitched battles with the more retro, motorcycle-riding, leather-jacketed rockers. A DIY teenage underworld had evolved so while The Rolling Stones sang "Mother's Little Helper," English mods dealt the "little yellow pills" on a thriving black market, and bands like The Who and The Move made themselves embodiments of pill-head triumph over hunger, sleep, orgasm, and reality.

The British mods had started out in the late 1950s and early 1960s, as a small, self-appointed elite who called themselves not "mods" but "modernists," and spent their time hanging out primarily in anonymous late-night clubs in London's West End. Their music was strictly the kind of modern jazz in which cool had replaced be-bop, and they looked somewhat askance at anything so crass as rock & roll. They borrowed their suits from the perfect style of Miles Davis, their shades from Ray Charles, and their porkpie hats from Thelonious Monk, but their pills were strictly Smith, Kline & French. Although almost exclusively heterosexual, the modernists cultivated effeminacy, some going as far as mascara and eye shadow. Being so few in number, they attracted little attention except the odd article in some up-market glossy magazine, and it really wasn't until large numbers of working-class youth aped a more robust, rock & roll version of their look—and also their taste for amphetamines—that the word "mod" was coined, and both the media and law enforcement began to take notice.

Although the British authorities, like their American counterparts, attempted to restrict the flow of pills, by crafting new anti-amphetamine legislation and putting pressure on doctors to cut down on the easy availability of the most popular pills, it was both haphazard and ineffective. Too many upright citizens, although they would never admit that they had such a terrible thing as a drug habit, took amphetamines of one kind or another on a daily basis for a variety of both real and spurious reasons. Also some types of pills were made harder to obtain than others. Drinamyl, the mix of amphetamine and barbiturate, was all but taken off the market, but the girls in the typing pool found it fairly easy to obtain prescriptions for Dexedrine spansules, time release capsules filled with delayed action micro-pills know as "green and clears," ostensibly either to counter fatigue or as a diet aid, but really to provide the same buffer against the boredom of hours pounding out mind-numbingly dull business letters. These, however, were scorned by rock & rollers since they provide a prolonged but mild high, instead of the faster hit of the famous yellow pills.

Many rock & roll bands toured Europe on a regular basis, and the legal availability of speed varied quite radically from country to country. Italy and Spain were notably lax, while Britain and France attempted to keep amphetamines down to at least a dull roar. (Although rock & roll bands did not tour in Spain until after the 1975 death of the fascist dictator Generalissimo Francisco Franco.) West Germany had a fairly restrictive policy towards any kind of speed pill, but with so many US military stationed on its soil to whom speed was still readily available, the Germans had trouble keeping it under control.

When police raided Redlands—Keith Richards' country home—in 1967, the charges brought against Mick Jagger were for possession of amphetamine, a controlled substance, without a prescription. Jagger claimed, however, that he had bought the drugs as airsickness pills from a vending machine at Rome airport, where the amphetamine content was perfectly legal. Unfortunately, this cut no ice with Judge Leslie Block who was determined to make an example of the notorious rock & roll band. Judge Block sentenced Jagger to six months in jail, and Keith Richards to one year for permitting his house to be used for the smoking of hashish, a holdover from an arcane Victorian statute used to curb the spread of opium dens in the 1890s. Had it not been for a public outcry and a scathing editorial by the editor of *The Times*, Britain's leading newspaper, titled "Who Breaks a Butterfly on the Wheel," both Stones would have done the time. Instead, on appeal, Jagger's sentence was commuted to a conditional discharge, and Keith's guilty verdict was quashed altogether.

That two of the Rolling Stones walked away from a sensational drug bust, however, did not mean that any tide had turned, or that the authorities on either side of the Atlantic were any less anxious to clamp down on what they saw as the scourge of drugs. Part of that clampdown was to permit less and less legitimately manufactured speed from reaching the streets. Again, though, as in the United States, when pills became harder to obtain in the United Kingdom, the outlaw manufacturers took over to service the undiminished demand. By the early 1970s, even the yellow SK&F Dexedrine were becoming an increasingly rare item, and something new was rapidly appearing in the pubs and clubs where speedfreaks hung out—a white powder of dubious provenance called amphetamine sulfate.

Plainly a Do-It-Yourself (DIY), bathtub-product amphetamine sulfate varied wildly in quality. Usually snorted through a straw or rolled up banknote in the manner of the much more expensive cocaine, some sulfate seemed reasonably pure and painless, while other batches burned like hell, and came with a disturbing smell of the kind of raw chlorine used to clean public toilets. This new form of speed often proved closer to nasty than drug-culture romantic, and about the best things that could be said for it was that it worked and the supply never ran short. No one quite knew the origin of amphetamine sulfate, and since it was highly illegal and seemed to have a definite connection to outlaw motorcycle clubs, no one really liked to ask. One thing was for sure, amphetamine sulfate had obviously never seen the inside of anything approaching a properly constituted laboratory, or been subjected to anything approaching quality control. Some claimed it was being made in Switzerland, from filched ingredients misappropriated from the massive Swiss pharmaceutical houses. Others claimed that Holland, with its increasing toleration of recreational drugs was the country of origin, and a third theory was that it was being cooked in secret on former hippie communes in green and pleasant rural England.

This new amphetamine sulfate, mostly coupled with hashish and alcohol, carried street-level rock & roll through the dire days of the early 1970s, when all was corporate glitter and stadium bands high on coke, tossing TV sets out of hotel windows, driving limousines into swimming pools, and shooting Polaroids of groupies who believed they were celebrities in their own right. Amphetamine sulfate kept a hundred desperate bar bands on the road, much in the manner described by Hank Williams Jr. just a few pages back, "You can postpone that morning after for a hell of a long time, weeks in fact and also you could play the shows all night if you wanted to." It also energized their equally desperate audiences, with their flared jeans and Rod Stewart haircuts, the disappointed former hippies whose abstract perception of a 1960s revolution had never materialized. Amphetamine sulfate kept the hard-scrabble rock rolling through intermediate pioneer thrash bands like Motorhead, (whose name was a less-well-used, alternative, low-life term for speedfreak) all the way to the spawning of punk, and the ripped-jeans rise of what might actually be, for a Sex-Pistols minute, a new youth movement.

The punks embraced the use of amphetamine sulfate with fervor. Its homemade, nostril rotting, gutter-drug ambience matched perfectly with their torn T-shirts, safety pins through the nose, bondage jeans, and anti-intellectual anarchy. It went with the filth and the fury, the truculent resentment, and anonymous blow jobs in the graffiti covered walls of punk club toilets. Just as amphetamine sulfate was Dexedrine without the finesse, the amplified electric razor fury, and snarling jackhammer pounding of first generation punk was The Who or The Move with an equal lack refinement. Even punk bands with record deals (did someone say The Clash?) maintained their street-drug credibility with beer and sulfate rather than going the decadent, rock-star, penthouse route of primo Bolivian flake, and all the other trappings of success.

Unfortunately punk, with its instinctive talent for self-destruction, found that the perfect way to pull the brakes on the headlong sulfate rush was to start messing with heroine. Without wishing to apportion blame, matters in London were probably not improved by how, in the mid 1970s, Keith Richards was at the pinnacle of his reign as king of junkie chic, and Johnny Thunders, former guitar-player with the New York Dolls, a faux-Keith and pretender-to-proletariat version of the same crown, had taken up residence in the city, and was a walking instruction for any wannabe-devious smack addict. (Some said Thunders was in London because he had done the seemingly impossible and worn out his welcome in the New York City drug culture.) Whether punk's adoption of heroin was motivated by role models, curiosity, or just a simple impulse to be the most messed-up punk on the block, that drug, like amphetamine sulfate, was also in plentiful supply. One source was wealthy Iranians, getting the hell out of their country, anticipating the fall of the Shah, and the inevitable conquest of Iran by a theocracy led by the Ayatollah Khomeini. Some had liquidated their assets and converted them into industrial diamonds, but others chose dope as the medium for easy, if illegal, under-the-radar transfer to the UK. Some of this new Iranian-supplied heroin was so pure that junkies, accustomed to dope that was barely more than 10 percent pure, overdosed on the Iranian's merchandise because they had never encountered anything so pristine.

All we know for certain is that, by the late 1970s, drug use among too many punks was a two-sided coin, or maybe a speedball switchback, going up on amphetamine sulfate on one side and coming down with heroin on the other. The casualty rate was high, with broken bands, discarded ambitions, and abandoned hopes for a fresh cultural revolution. There were also deaths, the most notable being that of Sid Vicious of the Sex Pistols, who, after stabbing his girlfriend Nancy Spungen, in room 101 of Manhattan's Chelsea Hotel, took what could only be described as a suicidal overdose at the home of his new girlfriend, Michelle Robinson, with heroin scored from, of all people, his mother. Sid, thus, became another posthumous role model for aspiring degenerates.

Holly Woodlawn has recalled her speed-freak breakfasts as "methedrine, melba toast, and a strong cup of coffee." My own were more like a pint of Guinness, the only thing my stomach would endure, as, unshaven, Manson-eyed, and three days in the same clothes, I wandered grey dawns with Lemmy (who ultimately founded Motorhead) in search of friends still awake who would listen to our plans for fame and world domination by the following Tuesday. Our worst rambling scenario was that we would be trapped in the squares' rush hour, and a world that rapidly transformed itself into yet another insane Wally Wood/*Mad* magazine crowd scene, and I would have to drag myself home, swallow Valium, talk to the less than receptive cat, and then sleep for 14 hours. ●

"SPEED KILLS"

PUNKS LIKED NOTHING BETTER THAN PISSING OFF hippies, and that might be one more reason that they were so enamored of speed with a side order of heroin. A decade earlier, in the supposedly golden age of peace, love, and flowers, the junkie and the speedfreak were considered the lowest of the low. The fiction began to circulate that acid heads were somehow superior to speedfreaks. Ironically, a definite snobbery permeated the illegal drug culture, coupled with a hierarchy in which junkies were openly condemned, and speedfreaks—scarcely much better—had a reputation for not eating or sleeping, fucking for hours, or not at all, talking incessantly, concocting elaborate conspiracy theories, making weird notes and drawings, exhibiting multiple obsessive-compulsive symptoms, and increasingly verging on the psychotic.

The slogan "Speed Kills" appeared on T-shirts, buttons, and as graffiti on the walls of hippie neighborhoods. The truth, however, was that many of the flower power generation were using both acid and speed, (and pot, beer, cheap red wine, vodka and anything else that might be going) and for drug users to start forming exclusive clubs around their drug of choice was little short of absurd. As decades passed, the role of the speedfreak as some kind of Serpent in the Garden during the Summer of Love has become greatly exaggerated by commentators looking for easy answers for "where the counterculture failed." That demonic differentiation reached a level of total implausibility when cultural historian Charles Perry, on a 2007 History Channel documentary called *The Drug Years*, claimed, in all seriousness, that "there were no cats left in Haight-Ashbury in 1967 because the speedfreaks ate them." Even the most cursory examination reveals the tale as arrant nonsense. No contemporary record exists of vanishing cats in the Bay Area, and to imagine anyone with a speedfreak's attention span trapping, killing, skinning and cooking a wily street feline when it would be so much easy to steal candy bars from a convenience store is nothing short of mind boggling. By telling such a preposterous story, Perry raises the suspicion that he is borrowing the hackneyed piece of racism about Chinese restaurants, and applying it to speedfreaks.

While not being kitty-eating zombies, though, junkies and speedfreaks did tend to cause more of their fair share of problems in major drug consuming cities like New York, London, San Francisco, and Amsterdam. Junkies stole to maintain their habits, while speedfreaks could be paranoid to excess and wholly irrational, and, of course, both lacked much that might be desired in matters of personal hygiene. Acidheads, on the other hand, were far cleaner, more metaphysical, and rarely prone to violence.

Acid—lysergic acid diethylamide, or LSD-25—was first synthesized by the Swiss chemist Albert Hofmann in the Sandoz (now Novartis) laboratories in Basel, Switzerland, but the powerful psychedelic that had so fascinated the spooks at MKULTRA had come to the streets of major western cities largely thanks to underground chemists like Owsley Stanley III, and had immediately cut a cultural swath in the budding counterculture. Promoted as an avenue to enlightenment by former Harvard psychology lecturer Timothy Leary, and the outlaw crew known as "Ken Kesey and his Merry Pranksters," (whose pranks were funded by the proceeds of Kesey's novel *One Flew Over The Cuckoo's Nest*) large sections of the underground community began to treat acid as a sacrament rather than an unusual and maybe insight provoking recreational drug. (Although some claimed that the whole phenomenon of San Francisco in 1966–'67 was really orchestrated by the CIA to see what might happen if LSD circulated on a citywide scale.)

Through 1967, psychedelia flourished on all levels. Paisley fabrics, swirling, curlicued graphic art, light machines from the simple to the highly complex, often combined with fluorescent Day-Glo paintings, all became part of the acid inspired circus, along with embellishments borrowed from art nouveau on one hand and eastern mysticism on the other. New kinds of nightclubs, ranging from the innovatively creative to the exploitative and tawdry, presented new bands with names like The Doors, The Jefferson Airplane, The Chocolate Watch Band or Pink Floyd were opening up not only in California, but in all of the major cities of the Western world, which inspired Frank Zappa—never a fan of recreational chemicals—to write the line "psychedelic dungeons springing up on every street."

But with methamphetamine and LSD proving themselves two of the most powerful mind altering drugs of the twentieth century, the inevitable dark side of human curiosity, sooner or later, had to ask what happens if the two were taken in tandem? Without doubt Sidney Gottlieb at MKULTRA had studied what cocktails of the two hallucinogens might do to the human mind, and found that results were, in most cases, a heightened sense of fear, advanced paranoia, and extreme—occasionally violent— anxiety at the resultant detachment from reality. For the most part, Gottlieb's experiments were conducted in the somewhat grim surroundings of a research lab or prison hospital, which could only serve to add an institutional edge to the almost inevitable horrors. Under more pragmatic and less clinical conditions, reactions were somewhat mitigated, but the consensus of opinion was that combining the two drugs was not a particularly smart idea. When an acidhead experienced the nightmare of a bad trip, the negative experience was frequently attributed to the acid being cut with speed.

Some less scrupulous denizens of the hippie underground observed, however, that, aside from generating a variety of horrors, at times, stretching all the way to Dr. Thompson's mythic "bat country," a mix of acid and speed could be used by any two-bit sidewalk Svengali to impose his will on the confused, the dislocated, the weak, and the stupid. During the summer of 1967, all of those types were flooding by the thousands into San Francisco and other urban centers with bohemian/artist/beatnik traditions. Psychedelic patriarchies and phony guru cults, run by suitably bearded, slightly older, hipster con men with barely plausible, mystical double-talk, assured their leaders of willing sex harems and panhandled coffers by dosing impressionable teenagers with acid, speed and anything else handy that sufficed to break down their traditional, middle-class conditioning and sexual inhibitions.

THE FAMILY THAT SLAYS TOGETHER

THE MOST celebrated of these manufactured faux-cultists was Charles Manson and his notorious Family who, by taking his convoluted philosophy—gleaned primarily from the Book of Revelation, the Beatles' *White Album*, and pulp/occult science fiction—all the way to serial mass homicide, guaranteed themselves, if nothing else, a permanent place on cable TV's History Channel. It is a matter of record that one of Charlie's basic techniques—essentially a psychedelic version of simple jailhouse/pimp psychology bolstered by pharmacopoeia—was to use acid to produce a sense that he was sole source of reality, and speed to induce paranoia of the outside world. His intent was to affect sexual reprogramming on his young and impressionable female followers, who were often on the run from their middle-class homes, and dissolve all remnants of conventional morality in order to indoctrinate them into Manson's mishmash

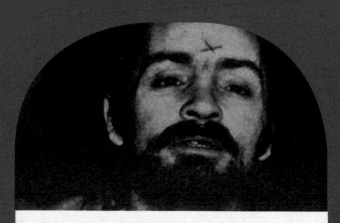

belief system of anarchy, the occult, and the world according to Charlie. Whether Manson's brainwashing was so thorough that his followers would kill at his command was wholly fact or a courtroom fabrication of Vincent Bugliosi, the Los Angeles County Deputy District Attorney who prosecuted and ultimately convicted Charlie, Patricia Krenwinkel, Susan Atkins, and Leslie Van Houten for murder and conspiracy in the Tate-LaBianca killings, may never be completely revealed. To prove conspiracy, Bugliosi had to succeed in convincing the jury that Charlie really did have some drug-induced messianic hold over his followers. ●

THE GREAT STRENGTH, AND ALSO THE FATAL WEAKness, of the hippie era was that it challenged and even broke a great many barriers. No one would pretend for a moment that the hippies came close to establishing a utopia, any more than they were able to turn the world, or even their neighborhoods, into replicas of an idyllic Maxfield Parrish landscape. For better and for worse, however, the poor did interact with the rich, black interacted with white, the unschooled hung with the educated, and maybe they all actually learned something in the process. (Even to read just Tolkien and Heinlein was better than not to read at all.) New perspectives were explored, even if it was all too frequently through a golden hallucinatory haze, or a ripped and jagged synaptic distortion.

The downside of this dropping of barriers and the partial dismantling of previous social structures was unfortunately coupled with an inability to come up with any functional replacement. Any speedfreak, with a few pills and enough beer to keep him lubricated, could expound at length about the counter-culture or the alternative society, but what they actually accomplished, for all their jive, was usually next to nothing except rushing out to score when the stash ran low. No one can deny for a moment that massive strides were made in the 1960s in media and the arts, and especially in music. Entire issues of underground newspapers were put to bed in frantic and grueling, 50-hour sessions, with editors, designers, and typesetters ragged on speed that had to be leveled off with beer, wine, or, green tea. Much happened, much was achieved, but, for the most part, the work was done by the minority, while the majority were content to just listen to Jimi Hendrix, read *The Fabulous Furry Freak Brothers*, laugh at Robert Crumb, or attempt to decipher the rainbow pages of the *San Francisco Oracle*.

When Aleister Crowley wrote his Law of Thelema, *"Do what thou wilt shall be the whole of the Law,"* it may have been grand, post-Victorian, rebel rhetoric, but it was hardly the basis for an entirely new revolutionary society. *Do what thou wilt* unfortunately applied equally to both the most gentle and well-meaning flower child, and a whole host of thieves, lowlifes, petty criminals, exploitative hustlers, and cut-price megalomaniacs. They only had to grow their hair and put on the costume, just like Charlie Manson had done when, after being released from the Federal Correctional Institution, Terminal Island, in Los Angeles, he made his way to San Francisco, arriving just in time to find flower power in full bloom. Like wolves in freaks' clothing, the ill-intentioned infiltrated a culture largely composed of unsuspecting sheep. An added advantage was that a high-profit and medium-risk drug culture was already in place to provide an infinite number of deals, scams, and rip-offs.

Many of the kids who had run away to join the scenes in cities with established bohemian enclaves lacked even enough street smarts to recognise when they were being suckered by criminals on the make. Twenty years earlier, the same characters might have been recognizable as the bad guys in double-breasted pinstripe suits, fedoras, black shirts, and white ties, but, in beads, buckskins, and bell-bottoms, they were taken at face value, until the boys from the suburbs found themselves relieved of their money and what was left of their worldly goods, while the girls might be turned out, stripping or turning tricks under the guise of "free love."

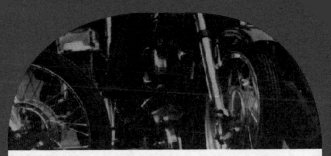

JUST ANOTHER MOUSE IN THE CAGE

DR. DAVID SMITH is a physician who has lived in San Francisco's Haight-Ashbury for 47 years. He opened the first Haight-Ashbury free clinic 40 years ago in response to a wave of drug-using young people who were moving to the city as part of the 1967 Summer of Love. Marijuana and LSD were a large part of the culture that was loosely united by music, art and opposition to the Vietnam War. By the end of that summer, Smith said his clinic was treating more and more young people for the effects of another drug: methamphetamine, made at the time by members of the Hells Angels Motorcycle Club and known on the street as speed. Unlike the peace-loving hippies high on pot, speedfreaks could be so violent that Smith had to treat them in rooms separate from his other patients. The clinic began the "Speed Kills" campaign that summer to discourage people from using the drug, a stimulant closely related to amphetamine. While many look back nostalgically at the 40th anniversary of the Summer of Love, Smith remembers it ending with heartache and violent disillusionment. Methamphetamine's violent effects were no surprise to Smith, who began his research into methamphetamine after hearing reports of the violent effects of diet-pill abuse in the so-called bohemian culture or Beat Generation. Smith focused on the drug in his 1965 thesis, in which he studied the effects of meth on caged mice, which normally are peaceful enough to groom one another. A mouse on meth, he discovered, interpreted grooming as a violent attack, usually prompting a fatal fight. "When all the violence hit, I thought, 'That's just like my mouse cage.'" ●

—*North County Times*, 2007

IF NOTHING ELSE CAN BE SAID IN FAVOR OF THE Hells Angels Motorcycle Club, they never attempted to disguise themselves as anything other than what they really were. Their colors, the winged death's head patches on the backs of their sawn-off Levi's jackets, distinguished them as outlaws in no uncertain terms. The relationship, especially at first, between the 1960s counterculture and the Hells Angels was decidedly ambiguous. Many romanticized them as some hipster version of a warrior caste, an odd hippie recreation of the Victorian noble savage concept tailored for the 1960s. To a certain degree, this attitude was reflected in the late Dr. Hunter S. Thompson's first book, *Hell's Angels: The Strange and Terrible Saga of the Outlaw Motorcycle Gangs*, first published in 1966. The idea was taken much more seriously by the Rolling Stones, who supposedly hired the Hells Angels in some protective or security capacity for a $500 donation to the club war chest and all the beer they could drink, when they played their hastily assembled, and now notorious, free concert at the Altamont Raceway near Livermore, California, on December 6, 1969.

Although debate continues to this day as to exactly what the Angels' intended function was at the show, many of them, especially neophyte "prospects," once drunk and stoned, and through the extremely long day, almost certainly speeding, began acting as the Stones' personal storm troopers. The resulting violence culminated in the stabbing and beating death of a man in a lime-green pimp suit named Meredith Hunter, who was seen (and caught on

film) swinging a long-barreled revolver and possibly looking to take a shot at Mick Jagger. The Stone's only previous
experience had been earlier in the same year with fledg-
ling, and much less violence-prone British bike clubs at a
similar concert in London's Hyde Park, and even that had
taken a degree of background negotiation on the part of
the London rock & roll/underground community to make
sure peace was maintained.

The Stones, before they hired the Angels as their faux-
romantic praetorian guards might have consulted more
closely with the numerous hipsters who had been in somewhat closer proximity to the club's members when they
were drinking and drugging, and knew they had a collective hair-trigger temper, a finely tuned sensitivity to insult,
and propensity to break heads first and ask questions later
or not at all. Even the good Dr. Thompson, after working
closely with the Angels on his book, still fell victim to a
serious stomping. The Stones would also have learned that
the Angels had a dangerously protective attitude towards
their Harley-Davidsons, and woe betide he or she who
might touch them without permission, and that they also
embraced the brawlers motto: "All on One—One on All."

Three years before Altamont, if only to preserve the
peace at their Acid Test promotions, Ken Kesey and his
Merry Pranksters had formed a truce—almost an alliance—with the Angels, who came to the events knowing
drugs and hippie girls were part of the attraction. Once
they were there, little could be done except accept them,
but Kesey and his house band, The Warlocks, later to become The Grateful Dead, managed with some degree of
success to impress the Angels that maybe cooperation with

this new phenomenon of acid freaks might be more to their advantage than boot-stomping hostility. The Dead had, unlike the Stones, had the Angels handle security at their shows without any kind of incident or mishap.

Down the pike, however, the Kesey-created détente between the hippies and the Hells Angels had an unexpected, but significant result. For the next decade or more, the Hells Angeles would control the California methamphetamine trade. ●

SPEED IN THE PEOPLE'S TEMPLE

CALIFORNIA, and the Bay Area, more or less in the wake of Altamont, saw the inception of one more amphetamine-related disaster, and, in this one, the body count was way higher. At the start of the 1970s, the charismatic and left-leaning preacher, the Rev. Jim Jones, who founded what amounted to a religious sect that he called the People's Temple in Indianapolis, moved on to bigger things in San Francisco, where the Temple formed a powerful political/religious coalition of poor whites and blacks and made important connections to the liberal city administration of Mayor George Moscone and Supervisor Harvey Milk. By the mid-seventies, however, stories were circulating that Jones, who had a taste for hair and sunglasses similar to that of Elvis Presley, was taking large daily quantities of prescription amphetamine, and that his mental health had started to deteriorate. Jones became increasingly paranoid that the

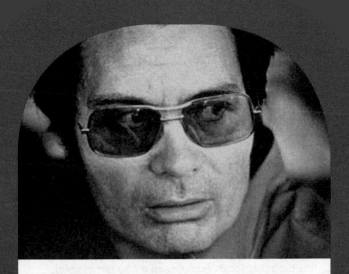

CIA was about to conduct some kind of vendetta against him. Accordingly—or at least according to Jones' logic—he moved the entire Temple in 1977, with close to 1,000 followers, to a jungle plantation he had created three years earlier in the former British colony of Guyana, where he believed he could establish a Utopian religious commune.

In Guyana, though, instead of finding an idealist refuge, Jones' paranoia grew worse. He was seemingly having regular shipments of speed sent from the US for his own use, and possibly that of others in his inner circle, plus large quantities of barbiturates, supposedly to keep his followers docile and in line. Rumors of abuse, beatings, and starvation in the Jonestown commune began to filter back to the United States, and a fact-finding group led by Congressman Leo Ryan went to Jonestown to investigate. This visit is accepted as the final factor that fed into Jones' speed-distorted imagination, and pushed him over the edge, convincing him that a biblical apocalypse was at hand. On November 18, 1978, Jones' followers machine-gunned Ryan and his party to death as they were leaving Jonestown in two light planes. After these killings, Jones and some 915 victims committed mass suicide by drinking Kool-Aid that was laced with cyanide.

That might have been the sorry end to the story, had not, as months passed, odd facts floated to the surface that didn't quite fit with the generally accepted line, and almost hinted that not everything was the product of Jones' over-fueled paranoia.

A full-blown conspiracy theory was underway that latched onto the fact that, in the week after the mass suicide, George Moscone and Harvey Milk were murdered in a seemingly unrelated incident. More twists were added by a Guyanese coroner's report, which received virtually no coverage in the US media, totally contradicted the idea of mass suicide, and stated clearly that the majority of victims had either been shot, or injected with lethal toxins, and that only two had poisoned themselves.

Far from being afraid of the CIA, the theorists claimed that Jones maintained a number of solid links with the agency via the notorious CIA torture expert Dan Mitrione, and an evangelical media group called World Vision, that many claimed was a CIA front, and was alleged also to have links to John Hinckley, who tried to assassinate Ronald Reagan, and Mark Chapman, who murdered John Lennon. The fevered supposition was that Jonestown was really a nightmare behavioral CIA experiment, which calls for massive paranoia within paranoia, but such can be the case when speed and the intelligence community are shaken not stirred. ●

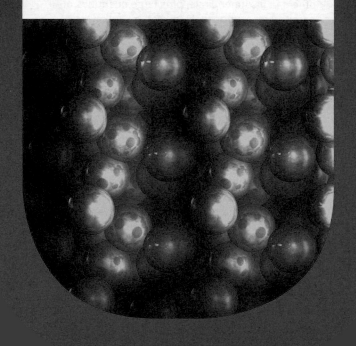

SPEED OF ANGELS

ACCORDING TO THE MOST ENDURING AND WIDE-spread of legends, the Hells Angels Motorcycle Club was founded in 1948 in Fontana, California, and some accounts claim the title was borrowed from the nickname of the US Air Force 303rd Bomber Group, although others insist the club was named for *Hell's Angels,* the Howard Hughes 1930 epic movie of World War I aviators that starred Jean Harlow and Ben Lyon. Ralph "Sonny" Barger, founder and president of the Oakland chapter (who might well be believed), describes the origins of the club as being more haphazard than most pop culture historians tend to imagine, and the early chapters of the club, most notably in San Francisco, Gardena, Fontana, and other Californian towns, were formed independently of one another, with the members initially unaware that any other Hells Angels clubs existed. A third account places the clubs origins in San Francisco in 1953, where they were formally named and organized by Rocky Graves, and were a direct successor to a gang known as either The Pissed-Off Bastards, or the Booze Fighters Motorcycle Club, who were largely responsible for the notorious Hollister riot of 1947.

The Hollister riot and a subsequent sensational account in *Life* magazine recounted, complete with equally sensational photographs, how a Fourth of July weekend motorcycle rally in the small town of Hollister, California sponsored by the American Motorcyclist Association, ran amok after some 4,000 bikers, girlfriends and hangers-on showed up—far in excess of any expected crowd—resulting in the town being overrun by rowdy bike fans who slept and partied in the streets and parks, and, at times, fell to fighting and wild disorganized bike racing. About 50 people were arrested, mostly for public drunkenness, lewd behavior, reckless driving, and disturbing the peace. A further 60 were injured, three seriously. The *Life* article in turn inspired the Marlon Brando movie *The Wild One*, and the black leather image of the outlaw biker was forever engraved on the public consciousness.

In the hope of restoring some kind of dignity and respectability to their members, the AMA issued a statement to the press in the wake of Hollister that "the trouble was caused by the one percent deviant that tarnishes the public image of both motorcycles and motorcyclists." Even this had the opposite of the desired effect. The embryonic bike gangs like the Booze Fighters, latched on to the term, referring to themselves as "one-percenters." It was even celebrated by a proudly worn jacket-patch on which a figure 1 and a % sign were enclosed in a red diamond.

True organization really only came to the Hells Angels in 1955 with 13 charter members, and Frank Sadilek, who designed the current death's head logo, serving as president. How exactly the Hells Angels became speed kings of the west is not exactly clear. In his 1967 book, *Freewheeling Frank*, Frank Reynolds, secretary of the San Francisco Chapter, writing with poet Michael McClure, talks about his own speed use of what he calls "geezing crystal" but seemingly does it in secret because the use of speed is seriously frowned on by his brothers in the colors. Even the fact that Reynolds had written a book, and was spending time with the intellectual likes of McClure and Lawrence Ferlinghetti, made him somewhat suspect with the club, and so he would hardly admit in print that he and his comrades in the San Francisco chapter were engaged in a felonious conspiracy.

As far as it can be calculated, the Hells Angels moved seriously into the speed business sometime between 1967 and the passing of the controlled substances act in 1970. At first it was a matter of buying/selling pills and arranging the odd drug store heist, but before long, the full potential of speed dealing started to be realized, and with the objective of monopolizing methamphetamine distribution in the entire Bay Area, the Oakland Angels began making their own meth. The formula was extremely simple, and the only real drawback was that meth cooking created a foul smell, and thus could not be done in any urban area. The Angels, however, had more than enough resources to set up makeshift rural labs to produce the merchandise.

While it may seem a tad absurd to look for positive benefits in a wild and woolly outlaw motorcycle club gaining a virtual monopoly on a powerful and illegal drug with frequently bizarre side effects, the Hells Angels at least kept the manufacture and distribution under a semblance of rough and ready control. Speed was always too unpredictable for the Italian mafia, and with the possible exception of some Detroit mobsters, they wanted nothing to do with either its dealers or customers. The Dons in New York, Miami, and rest of the Eastern seaboard saw no percentage in involving themselves in a highly unpredictable trade based in the wilds of California, run by heavily armed, unshaven cowboys on chopped-hog motorcycles. On the other hand, Mexican gangs on both sides of the border would have been delighted to carve themselves a piece of the lucrative West Coast speed trade, but for years, the Angels, and the other biker outfits like the Gypsy Jokers, with whom the Angels formed on and off alliances, were able to keep them at bay. In addition, the Angels were easily able to run off any independent amphetamine entrepreneurs who entertained the idea of usurping the Angels by going into business on their own.

By the early 1970s, the Hells Angels had such a lock on the speed traffic that they were able to spread it not only into the heartland of the United States, setting up chapters in some 23 states, but established what amounted to franchises in other countries. According to the *Vancouver Sun*, by the mid 1970s Canada had more Hells Angels members per capita than any other country, including the United States, and the club might have assumed more power had they not been challenged by native Canadian gangs like the Grim Reapers and Los Bravos, who, in a loose alliance, kept the Hells Angels from assuming dominance in the prairie provinces. At around the same time, the criminal intelligence section of the Royal Canadian Mounted Police who fulfill approximately the same function as the FBI in the United States, credited their Hells Angels with being Canada's largest volume methamphetamine dealers. Similar reports were also being filed in London by the Metropolitan Police Drugs Squad, and a scarcely believable Swiss Angel chapter was reputed to be hijacking truckloads of the raw materials used to manufacture speed from the vast Swiss pharmaceutical industry.

The Angels even managed to maintain a certain crude quality control over their product, if quality control is possible in a manufacturing process that includes toxic ingredients like ammonium nitrate, Red Devil Lye, and Liquid Fire drain opener. For a long time, the bikers' major ingredient was phenyl acetone (P2P), a chemical mainly employed to clean swimming pools, but the Feds countered this in 1979 by classifying P2P as a controlled substance. It was a dumb move on the part of the government, since the new restriction had unintentional and unfortunate consequences. The Angels and other meth makers began substituting ephedrine for outlawed P2P. Producing meth with ephedrine was easier, cheaper, and yielded a more powerful product. It was also where the chickens came into the picture.

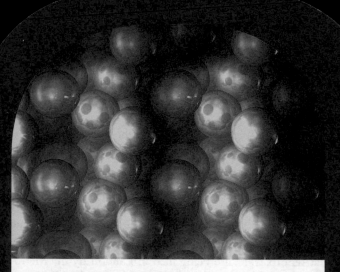

CONTROLLED SUBSTANCES

THE TIMES of shock wave and upheaval that brought the 1960s to a close were also when corporate amphetamine production began to be seriously curtailed, and the familiar pills and capsules (and the occasional ampoules of pure intravenous methedrine) began to vanish from streets and drugstore. The Controlled Substances Act of 1970 placed serious legal restrictions on any drug that matched the following criteria:

(A) The drug or other substance has a high potential for abuse.

(B) The drug or other substance has a currently accepted medical use in treatment in the United States or a currently accepted medical use with severe restrictions.

(C) Abuse of the drug or other substances may lead to severe psychological or physical dependence.

Clearly speed qualified for control in all categories, but unfortunately for the legislators, who wanted to outlaw all amphetamines as part of Richard Nixon's much heralded War On Drugs, one fact became clear to anyone in the underground who was interested. Speed was not especially difficult to make, and required no advanced chemistry, as was the case with acid. ●

THROUGH THE SECOND HALF OF THE TWENTIETH century, the Western world was eating more chicken than ever before. Hens no longer strolled the barnyard. Poultry was raised to be finger-lickin' good in vast factory-farm battery houses the size of aircraft hangers, with millions of birds racked as in some avian matrix. Breathing problems were endemic in these fowl mills, and feed was heavily laced with antibiotics, steroids, and bronchodilators, including ephedrine. One former biker described just how easy things were back in the days when outlaw speed went down on the farm. "If you couldn't steal a 50-pound drum of chicken ephedrine, you could buy it in an agriculture supply store. The cops didn't give a fuck about agri-chemicals or even ephedrine back then. You could also pick up ammonium nitrate, and maybe a shotgun, at the same place. Real one-stop shopping."

Even the Hells Angels couldn't make a good thing last forever. Although the Oakland Angels had tight grip on the Bay Area supply, they and the other chapters across the country and in Europe hardly had the manpower or organization for total world domination. Other biker groups, plus white supremacists like the Aryan Brotherhood and the Nazi Low Riders also moved into the meth trade. The word "crank" came into common use, and speed finally began to move in the direction of the trailer park, tattooed white-trash image that it enjoys today—what became dubbed the "all American high."

Although the Drug Enforcement Agency (DEA) and other government agencies like to rewrite history

to make the methamphetamine trade of the 1970s resemble a monolith of organized crime on a Harley, the
biker monopoly on crank actually kept it something of
a cottage industry—a dangerous and widespread cottage
industry, but a cottage industry all the same. Speed had
lost any kind of social cache (if it had any in the first
place). The disco hipsters in the flared pants had moved
on from speed to snorting cocaine, dropping Quaaludes,
and when things went bad, they could always turn to the
tired panacea of heroin. Methamphetamine continued to
be used, but was not considered a major problem. Speed
made a brief comeback with the event of punk rock, and
the new nose ring generation who snorted speed in order
to "slam in the pit," but then shot or smoked heroin to
calm down. Even so, in the world of international drug
cartels, biker speed was small change, and might well have
remained that way had not the DEA and FBI decided
they needed themselves some headlines and busted the
Oakland Angels. A report in *Time* from July 1979 makes
the move sound as though the Feds had taken down the
Gambino Family or the Medellín Cartel:

*18 Angels were arraigned in San Francisco on conspiracy
charges, and federal officials claimed in a 31-page indictment
that the gang trafficked extensively in illegal drugs, including heroin, cocaine, LSD and speed. They also contended that
gang members had murdered and threatened murder in order
to protect their share of the lucrative market.*

*According to the FBI, which began organizing a probe of
the Angels two years ago, the gang has between 250 and 300
members in the San Francisco area, with chapters elsewhere in*

California and in New York, Ohio and the Carolinas. "The investigation established that the organization existed for the purpose of violating the law," said Jerry Jenson, regional director of the U.S. Drug Enforcement Administration. "The club's bylaws clearly spell out that members will engage in distribution of drugs of a specified quantity and quality in order to remain members." By far the most popular drug sold by the Angels was methamphetamine (speed); investigators estimate that the club controlled up to 90% of northern California's methamphetamine trade. They indicate that the drugs were produced by the cyclists in five labs capable of turning out $160,000 worth of pills per day.

Most of the indicted Angels were arrested in a raid on some 30 locations throughout the Bay area. Among the apprehended were the gang's Oakland leader, Ralph ("Sonny") Barger, 40, and his wife Sharon, 29, a onetime beauty contest winner.

Officials seized a pound of speed and a slight amount of heroin, as well as a small arsenal of firearms, including some 1,000 rounds of ammunition.

Federal officers met with little resistance, but at the Angels' "clubhouse," a two-story stucco building in Oakland, they watched while 20 or so gang members roared off on their motorcycles. Oakland police were waiting two blocks away. According to the Drug Enforcement Administration, one Angel had a quantity of speed spilling from his shirt when he was arrested.

The trial of the Angels is set to begin in mid-August. Each defendant could draw up to 20 years. But even with convictions, says one federal official, 'there will be more of them out of prison than in, and you can't change years of a pattern overnight.'"

The high-profile campaign did not stop there. Through the 1980s and 1990s, the DEA, armed with The Racketeer Influenced and Corrupt Organizations Act (RICO) predicates and racketeering statutes, mounted a series of takedown campaigns against the bikers and neo-Nazis, disrupting what little organization they had left. In 1989, the DEA, for reasons known only to itself focused on San Diego as the heart of methedrine darkness. A raid on dozens of homes in San Diego County revealed a thriving methamphetamine industry. Hundreds of local, state and federal officers shut down 29 meth labs, arrested almost 100 manufacturers and seized 830 pounds of ephedrine, the drug's main precursor, in what, as usual, the DEA called the "single biggest roundup of meth manufacturers in the nation's history," and San Diegans woke up to the surprising news that their town was now supposedly the meth capital of the nation. The net result, however, was not the elimination of the demon speed—quite the reverse, in fact. The federal government handed the entire methamphetamine trade to the far more dangerously efficient Mexican underworld. ●

CHAPTER 7

SEX, SCIENCE, AND A LINE OF SPEED

"THE GUY WAS HIGH AS A KITE, AND, TO BE TRUTH-FUL, I have to admit that I wasn't much better. We'd been doing some kind of white powder and drinking vodka all evening, first with juice and then doing shots on their own. I suppose fucking had been the real goal all along, but when you're speeding there's so much else that's rushing through your mind its hard to concentrate on anything close to a goal. It took him a while to get a hard-on, but once the erection was there it stayed. And that was the problem. He simply couldn't come, but with the relentless determination of a goddamned speedfreak, he was going to try if it killed him—or me. At first it was a turn-on that he could just keep going and go-ing, although it did seem to be all about him and his orgasm, and I started to feel like little more than a means to an end. Plus I could sense a certain resentment. Maybe I wasn't doing *enough to help him. Remember that I was speeding too and when I'm speeding, I find it too fucking easy to feel paranoid and anxious, and that anything that might not be as it should be is all my fault. I wrapped my legs around him and did my best to help him get what he wanted. We changed position, I played with his balls, I said all kind of stuff to him that I don't even remember, but I suppose I was trying to get him off. Or maybe I was just trying to get him off me. The whole business was becoming a nightmare. The walls were closing in. This guy who had been sexy and funny and totally desirable was turning into a thing, all frustration and gritted teeth. A thing that just kept slamming into me and slamming into me. It was insanity. I was dry, I was sore, and I was getting damned fed up with it all. I used all my strength and was able to push him off me. For a moment I thought he was going to hit me. He looked fucking crazy, but then I think some shred of reality kicked in. He made this weird noise somewhere between a sigh and groan and rolled over on his side with his back to me, and started jerking himself off, angry, almost violent. I think I actually watched him for a few seconds. It was a so surreal. Then it occurred to me that he might want to start up again, and I grabbed my clothes and went and hid in the bathroom."*

The anonymous English woman is now in her early fifties, an ex-punkette, and she is actually recalling an incident from the 1970s, and the speed in question is the amphetamine sulfate of that era. Although today's crystal meth may be stronger, the patterns remain the same.

"I'm not saying that sex on speed was all bad, there were times when it could really be incredible. But, like so many other things that happened on speed, there was always the danger that everything could go completely off the rails. I

mean, that wasn't the only time when a man couldn't come, but it was the one that stuck in my mind. And then there were the times when the complete opposite happened. A boy would be speeding out of his mind and want to fuck me so bad, but he just couldn't get it up. Like the spirit is willing, you know? But the flesh won't work. And I'd suck him and play with damn thing forever, but...well...nothing."

On every level, amphetamine appears to be a two-way street on which things frequently don't go as planned, and its effect on the speedfreak's sex life is no exception.

"There was also something else about having sex on speed. I mean, it may have just been me, but, in retrospect, it always seemed like kinda impersonal. There are plenty of guys who, you know? They just want to stick their dick in you, and don't give a damn otherwise, but on speed, just like the endless conversations, its always about you, and the other person is just there for the ride, if you can understand that. Speed is the narcissist's high. You only want what you want."

Enhanced sexual desire and response are always on the standard list of the side effects of amphetamine and methamphetamine, but the lists fail to mention the complications that go with them, or that even the most rigorous academic or scientific study can hardly expect to be fully accurate when having sex while loaded to the gills on a highly potent and often hallucinatory drug can hardly be anything like subjective. Some women even claim that this idea of speed enhancing sex is a particularly male biased cliché, and that female speedfreaks have more of a sense of going along with their partner's heightened desires rather than wholly sharing them. They indicate that the drug creates such a sense of detachment from anything but self that it precludes any real intimacy, and that the sex act becomes a mechanical exercise, possibly enjoyable or maybe not. Former speed users also point out that it makes a whole lot of difference if both partners are high on speed or just one.

One former speedfreak recalled jokingly how, when she was high, she couldn't stop talking for long enough to be interested in sex. "I'm not saying that I didn't fuck on speed. Of course I did, often and with a lot of guys, and part of me really got off on it, but there was always this other area of my brain that was whirling around some other bit of the cosmos. To be absolutely truthful, my favorite thing when I was high was to have a man go down on me, just so I had this pleasant sensation to feel while I did something else. I could have happily read a book or done drawings while he was doing me. But that would have obviously pissed him off too much."

Another girl talks about the same sense of detachment, but with a slightly different, and maybe more extreme sense of detachment: "I swear there were times when I felt like I was watching myself doing all this stuff with some strange man. And even if he was my boyfriend, he was a strange man. All I could think was that it was just grotesque and weird. The whole sex business made no sense. I think sex on speed is much better for men than it is for women, but how can anyone tell? If you've done that much crank, you're close to psychotic anyway."

Psychotic or not, a 1992 Swedish study seems to bear out this girl's observation, and at least partially confirm the collected anecdotal comments. "Amphetamine users reported a higher frequency of intercourse on drugs with regu-

110

lar partners than did the heroin users. Sexual activity was claimed as the preferred activity on amphetamine by 51 percent of males and 20 percent of the females, and, of these, 23 reported that they became more sexually excited when on amphetamine, 21 reported intensified orgasms, and 23 reported that the drug prolonged intercourse and a greater interest in sex and greater frequency of intercourse."

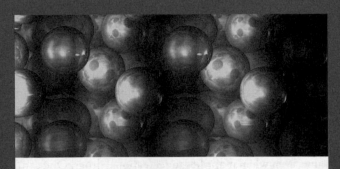

/KYROCKETED! THE MALE VIEW

"BEFORE ever trying meth, I had a normal, healthy sex drive. When I tried meth, my sex drive skyrocketed to the point where I was so horny, if a girl even massaged my shoulders I would start panting and trying my absolute hardest to get her to have sex with me. Sex on meth is fucking amazing and otherworldly: sensuality, response, drive, stamina and duration are all increased by a thousand-fold. When I stopped taking meth, sex didn't appeal to me anymore. Without crank, sex just seemed like a chore."

—Online ex-tweaker writing under the name of Rabid Lassie

NOT ALL WOMEN, THOUGH, SHARED THE OPINION that sex on speed is much better for men. A study conducted in Hawaii in 1997 quotes a 30-year-old woman talking passionately about sex and speed: "God what sex we had, Go! Go! Go! It gave me more courage. It made me braver. When a woman does a bit of crank she comes, climaxes. I had no idea it was two weeks! It was a lot of sex, listen to the stereo, more sex, do dope, talk, more sex, for two weeks. I could have gone forever, my kids missed me, days turned into nights and nights into days."

Perhaps she was part of the 20 percent as defined by the Swedish research, but no information was available as to her state of mind beyond the drug use, and, perhaps her real turn-on was the element of exhibitionism inherent in confessing to the researchers rather than her alleged weeks of sex, speed, and child neglect. Most of us have been conditioned to accept scientifically gathered evidence on its face value, even when it applies to recreational drugs. One can't help but wonder, however, about the scientific methodology used when yet another study equated human behavior with that of female hamsters dosed with amphetamine and reported—"sexually experienced animals responded sooner to amphetamine than did sexually naive animals. These data indicate that female sexual behavior can activate neurons in the nucleus accumbens and that sexual experience can cross-sensitize neuronal responses to amphetamine."

So if we are to believe that the sexually experienced, bimbo hamsters were more eager to fuck than their virgin sisters, how do we equate that with the human stripper who claimed she used speed to perform, because she found it enabled her to put a distance between herself and the audience: "A couple of toots would put me in a zone where I could fake anything, because the guys in the crowd became nothing more than cartoon characters and nothing mattered."

With all these perspectives on the same subject, who are we to believe: the researcher, the former punkette, the stripper on the chrome pole, the woman in Hawaii, or the promiscuous female hamster? I hesitate to suggest that the scientists should maybe try the drug themselves, at least once, to add an extra perspective to their work. Undoubtedly, they would say it would compromise their objectivity, but perhaps a certain subjective perspective might, now and again, add to the understanding of the human quotient in drug use, and provide more insight than the observation of hamsters. Lawmakers and those in authority tend to rely on studies and research—when it suits their political purpose—to frame legislation. Had all the research and study groups paid more attention to the motivation and social patterns of human beings, and less to the laboratory behavior of rodents, the catalogue of deadly errors and fatal mistakes that have been such a massive part and parcel of the twentieth and twenty-first century response to recreational drugs might have been greatly reduced. Nowhere were these errors more deadly than in the gay community in the second half of the twentieth century, where a crystal meth crisis ran headlong into the crisis of AIDS.

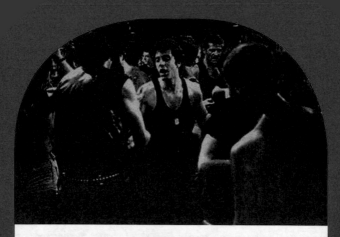

WITH HIS FOG, HIS AMPHETAMINE AND HIS PEARLS

"SOME of us use when we cruise because we find that meth heightens arousal and increases sexual stamina. There's also the delayed orgasm which makes play time go on and on and on. It's a big drag that impotence is a common side effect. This impotence is sometimes called crystal dick. You're sexually aroused but your cock won't cooperate; you can't keep it up or, even worse, get it up in the first place. Crystal meth may increase your confidence at the same time it lowers inhibitions. Under the influence, we might give in to our impulses and do stuff we might not otherwise have done. There's a big risk of HIV infection through unprotected sex, and perhaps more so while under the influence of meth. How come? Often enough, when we're zooming, everything we've been told, learned and practiced in terms of safe sex seems to be forgotten. And it's forgotten when we need it most because, when we're high, sexual activity and the desire for it increases like nobody's business. Some men who get fucked while they're high on speed are less sensitive to pain and may find themselves seeking out, asking for and having more aggressive sex for longer periods. Nothing wrong with an agro-fuck now and again, but without feeling all of what's going on, injury is more likely to occur and the risk of HIV infection is increased".

—Anonymous gay tweaker
writing online

SPEED HAS BEEN A DRUG OF CHOICE IN THE GAY community for about as long as speed has been a drug of choice anywhere, and for as long as there has been a recognizable gay community, mainly for the reasons stated by our anonymous gay tweaker—the sense of power and its potential for sexual enhancement. The Warhol Factory crowd and drag/drug queens like Holly Woodlawn, Jackie Curtis, and Candy Darling adopted speed. The only problem was that, in the closeted 1960s, to be both gay and a recreational drug user was to court a double whammy of public and official scorn. Indeed, most of the general public was totally unaware that there was a gay community at all. Although individual activists like Harry Hay and the Mattachine Society had been fighting for homosexual rights since as early as 1950, it wasn't until incidents like the Stonewall Riots in the summer of 1969 when, for five straight days, groups of gays, mainly men, and including a large proportion of drag queens, violently confronted the New York Police Department, after a raid on the well-known transvestite hangout, the Stonewall Inn on Christopher Street in New York's Greenwich Village, during which vice officers had used what club patrons considered unnecessary force and abuse.

Other similar occurrences had happened in preceding years, like the 1966 Compton's Cafeteria Riot of gay and transgender customers in San Francisco's Tenderloin district, when fighting broke out after police had attempted to arrest a group of rowdy drag queens. The Compton riot, however, failed to make the same headlines, and it was the protracted Stonewall clashes that became both a symbol and a watershed for the worldwide gay rights movement. Gays had never before acted together in such large numbers to forcibly resist police harassment, and they forced the public at large, and law enforcement in particular, to recognize that there was a not only a visible gay and transgender community, but that gay liberation was one more part of the same changing times that had given birth to movements like the Black Panthers, the Radical New Left, the women's movement, the anti-war protesters, and the hippie counter-culture.

The gays also quickly discovered that in this new and recognizable gay community—just as in the heterosexual hippie counterculture—all was not perfect. The gay community had its share of hustlers, criminals, and reckless drug abusers, and it definitely had its share of speedfreaks. Mostly they were viewed with the same disdain as in other underground cultures. They were noisy, frenetic, unkempt, and generally a nuisance. Most likely, if indirectly, they scored their drugs from the Hells Angels, but they were tolerated as basically going with the territory. (And they didn't eat cats.) The proportion of speed users may have actually been higher among gays than in other drug using underground communities because it was a group based wholly on a sexual preference, and a highly active sex life was a major factor for many of its members.

The new found sense of freedom that followed Stonewall, and the general feeling that gay men and women could finally stand up and be counted, was accompanied by equally new and open hedonism. In major cities like New York, and San Francisco, gay bars and discos, now largely free of harassment by undercover cops, went for the total extreme, and by the mid-1970s, the maxim "if you can imagine it, there's probably someone doing it right now," was never more true. From the half-naked bar boys of the super-exclusive Studio 54 to the leather-chaps-and-chains dress-code of subterranean bars like The Mineshaft, the party went full steam ahead. Speed of one kind or another provided fuel for the show, along with the more chic and expensive cocaine, the euphoric and inhibition-softening Quaaludes, (the sleeping pills that became so popular as a sexual prelude that bar-hoping singles wore gold replicas of them on chains around their necks) and the ever present amyl-nitrite poppers that were actually given away free like party favors at some gay bars. Speed even had its own nickname among gays. It was called "Tina."

As the gay dance and sex party roared on into the start of the Reagan 1980s, a brand new drug was added to the menu that was basically an inventive chemical modification of basic methamphetamine. The chemical name 3,4-methylenedioxymethamphetamine was far to unwieldy for any night club drug dealer or hopped up party boy, and at first, it was known by the easy initials MDMA, while some started calling it "psychedelic amphetamine" or "psychedelic speed." Ultimately the name "ecstasy," XTC, or even just X, would stick because it produced a touchy-feely sense of wellbeing and euphoria and easily overcame social reservations.

Essentially ecstasy was a kissing cousin of speed, but without the frenzy, paranoia, and jagged edge. Most users assumed that it was some new designer drug, based on methamphetamine, specially formulated for the late twenti-

117

eth century, but the truth was that MDMA had been around much longer, first patented by the German pharmaceutical giant Merck in 1912. It had, however, proved expensive to synthesize and had no real use. It was briefly tested by the US military in the 1950s under the code name EA-1475, but seemingly the Army could find no use for it although the results of this animal testing still remain classified.

MDMA was not resurrected until 1967, when it was tested as a psychotherapeutic by researcher Alexander Shulgin, after being made aware of it by Merrie Kleinman, a graduate student in the medicinal chemistry group he advised at San Francisco State University. At around the same time, small amounts of MDMA—at that time dubbed "the love drug"—appeared sporadically on the streets during the "Summer of Love" in San Francisco, but never caught the mass imagination in the same way as LSD. Nine years later, Shulgin would develop a new method of synthesis, and then introduced MDMA to Oakland psychologist Leo Zeff, who used the drug as an aid to talk therapy. Zeff, in turn, introduced the substance to hundreds of psychologists around the nation, and a number of therapists used it on their patients for enhancing communication, reducing psychological defenses, and increasing capacity for introspection until it was arbitrarily made illegal in 1985.

In yet another odd parallel between street and therapeutic drug use, MDMA again appeared on the streets at almost exactly the same time as Leo Zeff was first using it on his patients. This time, though, it wasn't ignored, and it very quickly became the preferred club drug for both hetero and homosexuals looking for a good time. Later it would become synonymous with the "rave" scenes of the eighties and nineties. In order to justify its illegality, stories of MDMA-related fatalities at raves began to circulate, not because rave attendees had overdosed or suffered any toxic effect, but because, supposedly high on XTC, they had danced for such extended periods in hot, crowded dance clubs, and they'd succumbed to dehydration, hyperthermia—literally, it was claimed, especially by the DEA, they had danced themselves to death.

X MARKS THE SPOT

(FROM A 2004 report of the National Institute On Drug Abuse [NIDA])

MDMA (3,4 methylenedioxymethamphetamine) is a synthetic, psychoactive drug chemically similar to the stimulant methamphetamine and the hallucinogen mescaline. Street names for MDMA include Ecstasy, Adam, XTC, hug, beans, and love drug. MDMA is an illegal drug that acts as both a stimulant and psychedelic, producing an energizing effect, as well as distortions in time and perception and enhanced enjoyment from tactile experiences. MDMA exerts its primary effects in the brain on neurons that use the chemical serotonin to communicate with other neurons. The serotonin system plays an important role in regulating mood, aggression, sexual activity, sleep, and sensitivity to pain. Research in animals indicates that MDMA is neurotoxic; whether or not this is also true in humans is currently an area of intense investigation. MDMA can also be dangerous to health and, on rare occasions, lethal.

For some people, MDMA can be addictive.

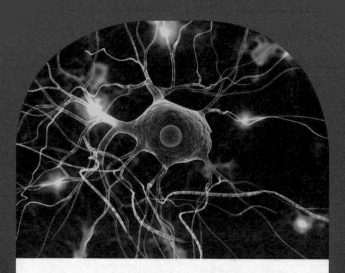

A survey of young adult and adolescent MDMA users found that 43 percent of those who reported ecstasy use met the accepted diagnostic criteria for dependence, as evidenced by continued use despite knowledge of physical or psychological harm, withdrawal effects, and tolerance (or diminished response), and 34 percent met the criteria for drug abuse. Almost 60 percent of people who use MDMA report withdrawal symptoms, including fatigue, loss of appetite, depressed feelings, and trouble concentrating.

Chronic users of MDMA perform more poorly than nonusers on certain types of cognitive or memory tasks. Some of these effects may be due to the use of other drugs in combination with MDMA, among other factors.

In high doses, MDMA can interfere with the body's ability to regulate temperature. On rare but unpredictable occasions, this can lead to a sharp increase in body temperature (hyperthermia), resulting in liver, kidney, and cardiovascular system failure, and death.

Because MDMA can interfere with its own metabolism (breakdown within the body), potentially harmful levels can be reached by repeated drug use within short intervals.

Users of MDMA face many of the same risks as users of other stimulants such as cocaine and amphetamines. These include increases in heart rate and blood pressure, a special risk for

people with circulatory
problems or heart disease, and
other symptoms such as muscle tension,
involuntary teeth clenching, nausea, blurred
vision, faintness, and chills or sweating.

These can include confusion, depression,
sleep problems, drug craving, and severe anxiety.
These problems can occur during and sometimes
days or weeks after taking MDMA. Research in animals links MDMA exposure to long-term damage
to neurons that are involved in mood, thinking, and
judgment. A study in nonhuman primates showed
that exposure to MDMA for only 4 days caused
damage to serotonin nerve terminals that was
evident 6 to 7 years later. While similar neurotox-
icity has not been definitively shown in humans,
the wealth of animal research indicating MDMA's
damaging properties suggests that MDMA is not a
safe drug for human consumption.

*(Let's also remember that NIDA never met a
recreational drug it liked.)* ●

UNFORTUNATELY, SOMETHING ELSE HAPPENED AS
the gay dance and sex party roared on into the start of the
Reagan 1980s. Two new and much more sinister sets of initials than MDMA would cast a long and deadly shadow.
These were AIDS and HIV. It's hardly the purpose of this
book to chronicle the history and the many speculative theories about the AIDS epidemic both global and domestic,
but when gay men and intravenous drug users began dropping dead of a new, unknown, and universally fatal disease,
one of the initial suspects was methamphetamine use (along
with ecstasy and amyl nitrite). Later research would demonstrate that HIV was a blood-born virus transmitted by either

unsafe sex, sharing needles, or a medical transfusion from a contaminated blood supply. Clearly speedfreaks who were shooting up now had to be ultra careful, but beyond that, amphetamine itself did not cause AIDS.

The connection between speed and AIDS might have stopped there, but, sad to say, it didn't. The psychological effects of all kinds of amphetamine, but especially those of the crystal meth favored in the gay community—the factors that made the drug so attractive in the first place—would start to pose a threat. The speedfreak, when high, enjoys a sense of omnipotence to the extent that the normal rules don't apply. One gay speedfreak told a researcher from the AIDS Foundation, "It frees your mind, especially if you are someone with self-esteem issues. It allows you to get to a point that you are better looking, you're better in bed, which encourages you to pursue someone on the dance floor or in the park." Reports started to come from San Francisco that speedfreaks were more prone to ignore the crucial need to use condoms when having sex with casual partners, and a government-sponsored report noted that HIV rates were three times as high among gay men who used methamphetamine. In another AIDS Foundation report one meth user commented, "When you are high and in that mindset, you really don't care. Doing it (without condoms) feels good. I want it to feel better. That is what I'm going to do."

Compounding an already dangerous situation, gay speedfreaks began to become mixed up with characters known as "gift givers," "bug chasers," and the practice known as "barebacking." A "gift giver" is an HIV positive man who gives the gift of HIV infection to another, while a "bug chaser" is the other side of the coin, the HIV negative man who deliberately becomes infected with HIV. The process known as "barebacking" is deliberate high-risk sex with disregard for HIV infection. In 2004, filmmaker Louise Hogarth made her documentary titled *The Gift* which chronicles this bizarre and apparently suicidal behavior. In one sequence, Hogarth visits a home where dozens of men are attending a "barebacking" party for unprotected sex, and in another, one of the films subjects, a 19-year-old called Doug Hitzel, recalls how he became a "bug chaser" in San Francisco. "Initially, something in me said you probably shouldn't do that, but after a while, I thought (becoming HIV-positive) would make me more popular. I ended up doing it once or twice. After a while, it became apparent people would like me if I didn't have a condom."

While audiences watched *The Gift* with a mixture of horror and fascination, they weren't aware that one more factor was in play. It wasn't until after the film was released that Hitzel, by then HIV-positive, admitted to *The New York Times* that he was high on speed during his bug chasing. "I don't really talk about the fact that there were a lot of drugs in my life at that point. I was into crystal meth, but I would never blame what I did on crystal meth, because I still fully take responsibility for my choices. But I think that at that point, honestly, when you are doing drugs and things, your health runs down. I was so sick. It messes with how you feel."

Doug Hitzel seemingly wasn't alone in his nightmare crystal meth madness, even before *The Gift* was released and the general public learned of gift givers and bug chasers, rumors had circulated, even making it as far as the straight world via the Showtime series *Queer As Folk*, of an underground network of what were known as "white parties." Ironically named for traditional high society, upper crust events where all the guests wear white, the attendees at these clandestine white parties usually wore very little except maybe a ball gag or a leather hood. The stories coming first out of Florida, then California and Nevada, and finally all over the United States, told of weekend, and even week-long, sex-and-drugs bacchanals, either at expensive private homes or specially rented spas or private hotels. At these events even the slightest concept of safe sex was totally thrown to the wind. These culminated during a legendary Easter in Palm Springs, attended by 7,000 gay men, that one wag described as "cesspools of reckless drug users having lots of risky sexual behaviors." The "white" after which the white party was named was the white of crystal meth. The increasingly plausible weight of second-hand accounts described the typical participants as wealthy older men who were able to not only reclaim some of the wildness of their youth, but could also pick up the tab, and attractive younger men from whom they could take their pick.

Journalist Eric Snider, writing in the Tampa, Florida *Weekly Planet*, interviewed a character going by the pseudonym of "Lloyd," now clean, sober, although unfortunately HIV positive as a result of his adventures on the white party circuit. In the course of the interview, Lloyd described how "there was a full SM dungeon in the guest room, replete with cages and all manner of paraphernalia. Strobe lights flashed, techno music blared and TVs flickered porno images virtually around the clock. Empty syringes, pot pipes and crack pipes littered the furniture. Sex toys were strewn all over. Naked men writhed in drug-fueled sextasy, anywhere, everywhere." Eric also recalls how, in the aftermath of a typical white party debauch, "(I had) pulverized myself on everything. I walked back to the hotel naked in boots, with a jock strap slung over my shoulder."

As though bug chasing and white parties weren't enough of a strain on the gay community, immunologist Madhavan Nair, at the State University of New York in Buffalo, claims that there is more than merely a social or behavioral link between speed and HIV. He sees a deeper biological connection right down at a cellular level, and believes that methamphetamine actually increases the risk of HIV infection. For reasons he has yet to discover, Nair claims the drug has a negative impact on a receptor in the body called DC-SIGN. Nair's explanation is complex but frightening. When speed use is prevalent among gay men, "The receptor is found on the surface of dendritic cells, a cell type that scavenges invading pathogens and presents them to infection-fighting T cells to activate an immune response." Nair discovered that immune cells exposed to meth make more of these receptors. "Unfortunately, in the case of HIV exposure, the additional receptors increase the risk of the virus infecting the T cells. The docking protein [the receptor] keeps the virus on the dendritic cell, and then it infects passing T cells." Thus unsafe sex and Nair's discovery of biological risks would appear to compliment and amplify each other. The distortion of the mind, and the cellular changes in the body conspire to create a deadly double whammy. Nair explains, "When people are using meth, they feel a superhuman feeling of safety, and their cells become more susceptible to the HIV virus. It's a dangerous combination."

The story of speed is beset by dangerous combinations, and not the least of these is that while the government and law enforcement spends millions of man hours and billions of dollars in a War on Drugs designed to eradicate methamphetamine, along with all the other recreational drugs that those in power—with no apparent consistency or logic—deem bad for us, hundreds of people have discovered that methamphetamine can be manufactured with little trouble by anyone who can follow a simple recipe composed of ingredients that can be found in any drug store, supermarket or hardware store. They also found that the process was not much more complicated than baking a cake, although with considerably more explosive potential. ●

THE DO-IT-YOURSELF FAST TRACK

THE DRAWBACK OF BEING A REGULAR CONSUMER of any kind of illegal drug is that one has to score. The drunk simply takes a walk to the liquor store, but the druggie is required to make more complex arrangements, and frequently finds him or herself in contact with numerous people with whom he or she has absolutely nothing in common except a shared taste in the same recreational high. In the case of the speedfreak, one tends to meet a whole lot of other speedfreaks, and these may not be particularly convivial encounters. I recall one time—to employ an increasing tired cliché—back in the day, when, while visiting the apartment of a London speed dealer to obtain a gram or so of the then-popular amphetamine sulfate. I happened to arrive just as another client was leaving, a talkative young man with very bad skin who seemed to be employed in some area of the punk rock business. As he made his departure, he happened to drop the gratuitous information that he intended to inject the speed that he had just scored. This information seemed to please the dealer about as much as a live hand grenade with the pin pulled.

"I really wouldn't do that, if I was you."

I felt the same, but since it was hardly my business, I said nothing, although I knew the sulfate from this source could vary wildly in quality, and frequently had a distinct, public urinal, chlorine reek, and a bad lot would seriously chastise the mucus membrane of the nose.

For some reason, this piece of good advice from the dealer made the punk rock needle fan decidedly defensive. "Why the fuck not?"

The dealer made a take-it-or-leave-it gesture. "Because I know the guys who make this stuff and they are not what you might call…" He searched for the right words, "…all that careful."

In Kevin Booth's stunning 2008 documentary *American Drug War: The Last White Hope*, one of the most blunt critics of current drug policy was Robert Steele, described in the film as an "ex-CIA Agent who after realizing that his job with the CIA was to protect the interests of huge corporations and not the American people, left and has now become a major thorn in the side of his former employer." Booth didn't hesitate to point out the arrant absurdity of federal and local law enforcement attempting to rid the country by judicial force of a drug that can easily be manufactured in any garage, outhouse, or trailer.

One fairly typical recipe for meth manufacture is published on the *totes.com* website in which an anonymous meth cooker, like some demented Julia Child, shows just how simple meth manufacture can be, and also how physically dangerous, and the writer does preface his description with the very basic safety warning—"You will be using dangerous chemicals while producing this shit. This is not a fucking game; this is not something you do for fun; you MUST know what you're doing." But he also boasts, "I have used this formula and made a 1/4 pound of some high quality shit."

The website recipe calls for 200 pseudoephedrine pills (Actifed, Sudafed, Suphedrine, etc.), one and a half cups of ammonium nitrate fertilizer, three cans of starting fluid, three AA Energizer lithium batteries, one bottle of Red Devil Lye, water, iodized salt, and one bottle of Liquid Fire drain opener. Another substitutes sulfuric acid and aluminum foil for the lye and drain opener. Other cookers recommend crushed aluminum beer cans. All the components in these hellish brews are the basic ingredients in what's known as the "Nazi method" of cooking methamphetamine. (So named, the writer explains, because "the Nazis used meth during WWII to make their troops super-hyper and CRAZY as FUCK. Hitler loved the stuff, which may be why he came up with so many amazingly BAD IDEAS.")

At this point, your author chickens out of describing the exact procedure to turn all of these assorted substances into crystal meth. To do so, as we shall later explain, is to run the risk of having the FBI, DEA, or some local district attorney all over the author and publishers asses. Suffice it to say that the sum total results in a bubbling brew that, once it stops bubbling, should be "given a stir and let it sit for 4 hours. After 4 hours CAREFULLY pour out the nasty liquid. You will see a lot of gunk at the bottom, that's all meth. Get it all out and let it dry. Once dry, it will be one big chunk of rock. You can crush it up into a powder form and sell it as crank (which seems to go farther), or you can break it off in small chunks and sell it as Ice (goes shorter but people LOVE ice). After you're done, you will have 1/4 pound of meth, which is 4 ounces. I sold 3 and kept one for myself." But the process, although simple, is seemingly fraught with pitfalls. The online instructor issues stern warnings—"wear a mask and gloves if you can; do it someplace remote; be careful of the sulfuric acid because that shit will eat you to the bone, and make sure there's not moisture in or around the bucket, or KA-FUCKING-BOOM!" The cooker ends with one last heartfelt safety warning. "Don't be a dumbass. KNOW WHAT YOU'RE FUCKING WITH!!!"

This simple internet recipe offers not only the prevailing attitude to the home cooking of crystal meth, but also the mindset of the cooker, who seems to consider himself part cowboy, part anarchist, and part high school chemistry nerd, and is clearly buying into the quasi-reality that the meth cooker has become, in this drug drenched society, a piece of modern American folklore. He or she is the contemporary equivalent of the old time moonshiner with a still in the backwoods, a fast car, and a healthy dislike for the "revenue men." Badly brewed white lightning could kill you, and so can DIY crank, but that doesn't seem to diminish the probably unhealthy fascination with either example of outlaw chemistry. The news media, especially the local news, recognizing what will sell to their viewers, positively delight in the discovery of meth labs with pictures at eleven. Insatiable TV crews race to the scene each time an isolated trailer explodes and burns up on the badland edge of town, or cops in flack jackets and firemen in HAZMAT suits surround a bungalow in an outlying suburban slum. The commentary comes complete with words like "scourge" and "plague," and spokespersons for the DEA or local law enforcement issue dire warnings about how, unless stopped, crystal meth will be the death of America.

Movies like *Spun* and *Salton Sea* have shifted the dynamic from the sensationalism of media facts—or maybe factoids, as oft-repeated errors are accepted as reality—to the stuff of fictional legend. In *Salton Sea*, the mad amphetamine faux-scientist, played by Meat Loaf, reenacts the JFK assassination with toy cars and a cast of unfortunate chickens, while in *Spun*, Mickey Rourke plays a character called The Cook as a disreputable cowboy in a motel and tract home, psychotic, neo–Wild West.

In his 2005 book *American Meth*, Sterling R. Braswell makes the valid point that "the early incarnations of the methamphetamine street chemists were a far cry from the meth cooks of today. The former were nor only smart but arguably brilliant. Surely some must have learned their craft in the world of legitimate chemistry and pharmacology, only to lose their way experimenting with means and methods of brewing a wide variety of methamphetamines and what would come to be known by their eerily modern rubrics of "analogue," or "designer" drugs, such as MDE, MDA, MDMA, MDME... Their work had to take into account not only chemistry, but brain chemistry—scien-

131

tific considerations which had to come in line with legal and market place realities."

Unfortunately, the net effect of "legal and market place realities" has been to set the whole process of manufacturing speed on a downward course that, through the twentieth century, took it from the pristine and quality-controlled labs of Smith, Klein, & French to seedy motels and desert hideouts where the heavily armed madmen of popular imagination practice the "Nazi method" as earlier described, and preside over bubbling vats of lithium batteries and Red Devil Lye, in a sub-world where punk fantasy usurps a Jim Thompson novel. At no time has the concept of harm reduction ever entered the landscape of making or using amphetamine.

Harm reduction has never been popular in the United States. As the War on Drugs has dragged on for more than 70 years, few attempts have been made on anything but the most modest scale to address the problem of recreational drug use and abuse as a medical problem rather than a judicial one. All too often those who have advocated that both the drug user and society at large would be better protected by the decriminalization, the regulation, and the maintenance of a high purity in the drugs themselves, than by arresting and imprisoning users and suppliers, have been shouted down by the drug warriors as bleeding hearts bent on mollycoddling the evil addict. Some have even been accused of having far more sinister agendas that seek undermine the core values of the nation.

DO NO HARM

FROM THE Drug Policy Alliance, 2008:
Harm reduction is a public health philosophy that seeks to lessen the dangers that drug abuse and our drug policies cause to society. A harm reduction strategy is a comprehensive approach to drug abuse and drug policy. Harm reduction's complexity lends to its misperception as a drug legalization tool. Harm reduction rests on several basic assumptions. A basic tenet of harm reduction is that there has never been, is not now, and never will be a drug-free society. Harm reduction approach acknowledges that there is no ultimate solution to the problem of drugs in a free society, and that many different interventions may work. Those interventions should be based on science, compassion, health and human rights. A harm reduction strategy demands new outcome measurements. Whereas the success of current drug policies is primarily measured by the change in use rates, the success of a harm reduction strategy is measured by the change in rates of death, disease, crime and suffering. Because incarceration does little to reduce the harms that ever-present drugs cause to our society, a harm reduction approach favors treatment of drug addiction by health care professionals over incarceration in the penal system. Harm reduction seeks to reduce the harms of drug policies dependent on an over-emphasis on interdiction, such as arrest, incarceration, establishment of a felony record, lack of treatment, lack of adequate information about drugs, the expansion of military source control intervention efforts in other countries, and intrusion on personal freedoms. Harm reduction also seeks to reduce the harms caused by an over-emphasis on prohibition, such as increased purity, black market adulterants, black market sale to minors, and black market crime. Finally, harm reduction seeks to restore basic human dignity to dealing with the disease of addiction. ●

WE MUST ASSUME THAT LAWMAKERS, BOTH STATE and federal, were well intentioned when they devised the parade of restrictions and criminal penalties that have sought to curb or eliminate the manufacture, supply, and manufacture of amphetamine. To do otherwise would be to accuse them of the most onerous deviousness and corruption. (We can't have that now, can we?) Rather, we have to assume that those in power were simply, though seriously, mistaken, when all of their efforts to eradicate what they saw as the danger of amphetamines had a wholly reverse result. Perhaps Robert Steele, the ex-CIA agent referenced earlier, was waxing eloquent when he condemned the absurdity of trying to outlaw a substance that can so easily be produced by an amateur chemist in an outhouse. Unfortunately, even the most cursory hindsight demonstrates all too clearly that almost all of the measures taken to remove speed from the landscape of American drug use have only served to exacerbate the situation and make its presence more overwhelming.

The story would appear to be one of a constant substitution of ideology, and the illusion of winning the nebulous drug war, for common sense. In the beginning, bennies were bought over the counter, but the fear of unwanted and possibly detrimental side effects caused them to be restricted, and they were made legally unobtainable except by a prescription from a doctor. This created a situation in which most of the recreational amphetamine came from still manageable pool of pharmaceutically produced drugs that were the result of either over-prescribing or the occasional drugstore heist. On a pragmatic level, this might have been acceptable, but legislators argued that laws were being violated, and also they're avowed intention was to create a society free of all drugs except nicotine and alcohol. The police went to work, and on the street, the familiar Dexedrine, black beauties, and white crosses became increasingly scarce. While the pills and capsules became harder to find, the demand in no way diminished, and for the first time, bootlegged manufacturing began.

As we have seen, this initially came mainly under the control of the Hells Angels and other outlaw motorcycle clubs. While in no way overestimating the altruism of the biker, or suggesting that they had very much of a social conscience, they ran a tight ship. They discouraged competition and did maintain a crude level of quality, if only because they looked to stay in business for the long term, and hold on to their various territorial monopolies, something that would hardly be possible if they were delivering inferior product. Once again, a certain pragmatism might have suggested that the authorities, on the principle of keeping the speed trade down to a low roar, since it obviously could never be totally wiped out, might have accepted this as a form of status quo, and concentrated on combating the worse speedfreak excesses through education and making medical care available to those who needed it—in other words, harm reduction.

For a while, it actually seemed as though the low roar strategy was being adopted. DEA or local drug agents would bust labs when and where they could, but were hampered by the fact the Hells Angels primary ingredient—what was know as the precursor chemical—was the pool cleaning agent P2P, and P2P was totally legal both to purchase and possess. In order to bust a lab, instead of just chasing users and various levels of dealer on the supply chain, the narcs needed first to spot their cooker, then tail him until he picked up a consignment of equipment and chemicals at a chemical supply company, follow him to wherever the makeshift lab was to be set up, and then wait, hoping that, by a combination of estimate and informed guesswork, they could kick the door down at exactly the right moment. They needed to stage the bust when the meth was actually meth. If they arrived too early, they had nothing but a mixture of legal chemicals. If they came in too late the meth would be long gone.

Still believing the myth that the meth business could be finished once and for all, the DEA lobbied congress for a new weapon in their arsenal, and congress, in 1980, with absolutely no consideration of any future implications, outlawed the pool cleaner P2P by including it in Schedule II of the Controlled Substance Act. This briefly threw a spanner into the meth cooking business, and the DEA reported a brief decline in lab seizures. The outlaw chemists, seemingly having more forward-thinking ingenuity than the government, simply found themselves a new precursor chemical. Instead of the now illegal P2P, they began using the drug ephedrine in something called the hydriodic acid/ephedrine reduction method, which was, in fact, a simpler and more efficient process than the one that employed P2P.

Ephedrine is familiar to older asthmatics as a popular and widely used bronchodilator. It continues to be the active ingredient in nonprescription asthma cures both in pill and inhaler form, but over the years, has largely been replaced by the more efficient salbutamol and other more modern chemicals. It has also enjoyed popularity as a diet aid, can still be purchased through the internet, and is widely used in the agri-business as decongestant for poultry. The drug has a history going back some 5,000 years, as part of Chinese traditional medicine, in which the ma huang plant was employed under a whole multitude of circumstances as an all purpose stimulant. In the West, ma huang is know as ephedra, and is not only the source of ephedrine, but also its chemical cousin pseudoephedrine, that was, up until the crystal meth panic of 2004–2005, the principle ingredient of Sudafed and other decongestants. Most of the ephedrine used in the United States is manufactured in China where its production represents a huge and profitable export industry. China ships approximately 30,000 tons of ephedra each year at an estimated value of $13 million, which is 10 times the amount used by the Chinese.

Authorities quickly discovered that a major error had been made when P2P had been outlawed and the speed chefs had been forced to move on to ephedrine. Not only was the drug's molecular structure so close to methamphetamine that it made the conversion extremely easy, so easy, if fact, that totally untrained individuals were able to move into the meth production business. To add insult to irony for those in power, ephedrine also enabled cookers to turn out a cleaner and better quality product. The meth made by processing P2P was lucky to average 30 percent pure, but with ephedrine as the precursor chemical, the purity count rose as high as 60 percent. The first reaction by the DEA was to look for ways to make the sale and possession of ephedrine illegal, but the drug warriors quickly discovered that this would not be anything like as easy as getting rid of the low profile pool cleaner ingredient P2P. At approximately the same time that P2P was outlawed, ephedra was enjoying 15 minutes of fame as the wonder drug of health food and fad diet devotees, and was sold everywhere. It was available in various forms in health-food stores and via direct mail 800 numbers on late-night TV commercials, and even positioned beside the cash register at convenience stores as a quick pick-up. Live plants and seeds were also legally imported into the United States by exotic or medicinal plant dealers. This widespread use of ephedra made it much harder to place under any kind of blanket restriction.

THE ICE COMETH

IN THE LATE 1980s word began to come out of Hawaii, and the West Coast of the mainland United States, of a new form of methamphetamine that could be smoked, and keep the user crazy-high for up to two or three days, complete with audio-visual hallucinations, paranoia, and a tendency to uncontrolled violence. This supposed new form of speed was primarily know as "ice," although the name "glass" was occasionally heard, and even "shabu," the old Japanese 1950s nickname for Yakuza speed. Initially "ice" was pitched as being a brand new and highly exotic drug, supposedly developed in either China or South Korea, but shrouded in mystery. Ice was described in both media and drug-culture rumor as being essentially the speedfreak's equivalent to crack cocaine that was, simultaneously, enjoying its ghetto vogue—sponsored, we would later learn, by the Central

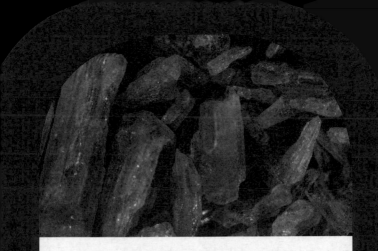

Intelligence Agency, Colonel Oliver North and the Iran-Contra conspiracy, through street-level middle-men like Freeway Ricky Ross, the kingpin who ran the crack epidemic in South Central Los Angeles, and who only discovered that he was fronting for the CIA after he was busted.

For a while, something of a panic reigned that ice would spread across the US and maybe on to Europe as the new "killer drug" to follow crack, leaving addicted bodies and broken lives in its wake. The panic was so great that it took a while for even experienced speedfreaks to figure out that ice was nothing more than basic methamphetamine in a crystal form.

This is not to say that smoking cheaply made crystal meth is in any way a good idea. In many respects it's a worse idea than shooting the stuff. It gives an instant hit that very easily becomes a seductive habit, and the direct effect of moving chemicals from the lungs to the bloodstream is very akin to shooting meth, except the dangers of taking absurdly massive amounts of the drug are far greater that either snorting the stuff or ingesting it orally—and even the needle-using freak might be deterred by the quantities of speed the smoker can inhale without knowing it. Further risks include having meth by-products crystallize in the lungs, and development of a toxic sweat condition that can cause serious skin rash and running sores. In many respects, the ability to smoke crystal meth had been a serious factor in all the horror stories of major meth epidemics through the 1990s to the present day. ●

THE FIRST MOVE TO PREVENT ACCESS TO EPHEDRINE by speed cookers was some legal slight of hand by the DEA and the Justice Department whereby the provisions of the Chemical Diversion and Trafficking Act of 1988 were used to bring ephedrine at least within reach of the Controlled Substances Act. Ephedrine and ephedra were not made illegal per se. Even though Ronald Reagan's Attorney General Edwin Meese had given himself the arbitrary power to outlaw any new drug he didn't like, even he and the DEA couldn't simply take a 5,000-year-old Chinese herbal remedy and declare it illegal. Instead, an order was issued that required all shipments of bulk ephedrine and single entity-ephedrine drug products be flagged by the government, tracked to the purchaser, and the legitimacy of its use investigated.

At around the same time, the ephedra fad began to wane. Anecdotal reports linked ephedra, especially when used as a diet aid, with heart palpitations, tremors and insomnia, and also dangerous levels of dehydration when exercising while using products containing ephedra. A 2003 RAND Corporation study, commissioned by the National Institutes of Health, called into question the safety of ephedra, and appeared to confirm fears that both ephedra and ephedrine were related to an entire menu of health problems. By this time, the US Food and Drug Administration (FDA) had also become involved and had announced its ultimate intention to ban products containing ephedra and its extracts. The FDA claimed its action was justified by health problems including some deaths. Horror stories began to circulate, and were followed by a rash of lawsuits. An Alabama jury ordered diet pill maker Metabolife International to pay $4.1 million to four people who suffered strokes or heart attacks after taking an ephedra-based appetite suppressant, while the families of a dead 28-year-old bodybuilder in Las Vegas and a dead 27-year-old Marine Corps officer in Florida sued Twin Laboratories Inc. blaming the deaths on the company's ephedra supplement called "Ripped Fuel."

Not everyone, however, bought the FDA's public pronouncements. Conspiracy theorists opposed to the War on Drugs denounced the FDA's increased scrutiny on ephedrine as nothing more than a smokescreen, created in cahoots with the DEA, to remove ephedrine as a methamphetamine precursor. The diet-pill industry admitted there might be some risk of side effects associated with using ephedrine as a diet supplement, and agreed that their products could certainly carry a warning label, but complained that an outright ban was wholly excessive. Then, in 2003, a Florida medical examiner linked an ephedra supplement to the death of Baltimore Orioles pitching prospect Steve Bechler during that year's spring training. The FDA had all the excuse it needed and immediately used the tragedy to prove its point on ephedra. The agency issued a fast press release, "Throughout America, there continue to be tragic incidents that link dietary supplements containing ephedra to serious health problems in consumers that use these products," and henceforth all products containing ephedra or ephedrine would carry prominent labels warning that they could cause heart attacks, seizures or death.

The American romance with ephedra was at an end, and the stage set for a total ban on the ancient herbal derivative, which came at the end of 2003 when the FDA announced plans to do exactly that, and on April 12, 2004, an agency rule prohibiting the sale of dietary supplements containing ephedra went into effect. Legal appeals were lodged, but by August of 2006, the US Tenth Circuit Court of Appeals upheld the FDA's ban on all ephedra products sold for human consumption, and that was that. Dieters and athletes with a taste for ephedrine products had either stopped using ephedra, had stockpiled enough supplies to keep them going, or were mail-ordering them from Canada which was still at least semi-legal. As one woman whose weight loss regimen included ephedra products remarked, "That's what Canada's there for." At the same time, the legal seesaw process had given the small time DIY methedrine cookers enough breathing space to stay a jump ahead of the authorities, and switch to a slightly different means of production and a slightly different precursor drug.

While the FDA had been going after ephedrine, the meth makers had moved on to what turned out to be an even more easily obtained basis for their product. Pseudoephedrine, the close ephedrine relative, was the basis of over-the-counter cold and allergy remedies like Sudafed, Actifed, and Nyquil that could be picked up in any drugstore, convenience store, or supermarket. It might have been somewhat suspect when an unshaven and somewhat dubious dude in a leather cowboy hat, engineer boots, and a Motorhead T-shirt purchased an entire case of Sudafed, but few minimum-wage checkout clerks were going to question the transaction. The War on Drugs was hardly their problem, and what were they going to do anyway when the purchaser snarled back that he was having "one fuck of a bout of flu"?

The DEA and local law enforcement weren't slow to see what was happening, and their response was standard. The media was alerted, yet another cycle of speed hysteria was initiated with unseemly relish. News items about meth yet again proved a boon to copy-hungry, small town newspapers and TV stations, who gleefully repeated horror stories of "addicts so high on meth that even a Taser won't stop them," described how "meth addicts believe that everyone is out to get them, even innocent strangers or inanimate objects," and once again rolled out ponderous editorial phrases like "the crisis of the new millennium." Even network news couldn't resist. In July of 2005, CBS ran a sob story on the "new generation of helpless victims"—the "meth orphans"—children who are taken from their parents after raids on home meth labs, and are "stretching an already strained child welfare system to its limit." On August 9, NBC schlepped out Drug Czar John Walters to underline the alarm over "meth orphans," and underscore the new "what-about-the-children?" spin in the propaganda war on speed. The hysteria wasn't only limited to propaganda. Some jurisdictions demanded that citizens buying cold cures be required to give their names, addresses, telephone and driver's license numbers to store clerks. Indiana was especially frenzied and state police claimed to have busted 1,500 meth labs, while North Carolina employed anti-terrorism laws to prosecute meth lab cases.

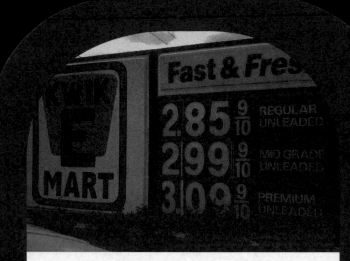

FEDS IN THE KWIK-E-MARTS

THE NORTHERN District of Georgia actually went after the store clerks. In a bizarre sting operation called Operation Meth Merchant, ex-cons and speedfreaks—usually as part of a plea deal—were sent out to rural Georgia Kwik-E-Marts to buy Sudafed, and make known their intention was to cook up a batch of meth. Operation Meth Merchant netted 49 convenience-store clerks and owners who were charged with selling materials used to make methamphetamine, and each faced up to 20 years in prison and $250,000 in fines. Federal prosecutors claimed that hidden cameras and microphones had caught workers acknowledging that the purchases were for cooking meth. As the cases came to court, the truth quickly emerged that all but five of the defendants were Indian immigrants (32 were named Patel, which made the rednecks very paranoid, but only indicated they came from the Gujarat area) and their command of English was purely transactional, less than that of Apu Nahasapeemapetilon of *The Simpsons* fame. Hajira Ahmed, whose husband was charged with selling cold medicine and antifreeze at their store on a back road near the Tennessee border, voiced the general confusion to a reporter from *The New York Times*. "This is the first time I heard this—I don't know how to pronounce—this meta-meta something." ●

IN AN ATTEMPT TO STANDARDIZE THE LAW ON A federal level, and maybe prevent more ludicrous grand-standing like Operation Meth Merchant, Senators Dianne Feinstein, D-CA, and Jim Talent, R-MO, cosponsored a bill requiring stores to sell Sudafed, Nyquil and other medicines containing pseudoephedrine only from behind the pharmacy counter. Consumers would have to show a photo ID, sign a log, and be limited to 250 30 mg pills in a 30-day period. Computer tracking would prevent visits to multiple stores. Meanwhile Pfizer, Inc., the manufacturer of Sudafed, introduced Sudafed PE in January 2006. Made with phenylephrine, Sudafed PE cannot be cooked down into meth. Retail pharmacists were dubious about the legal stampede to eliminate pseudoephedrine. One complained "Imagine you're in line and you're sick and getting antibi-otics and you have to wait behind three people who have to fill out a stupid log."

A worse problem was that hysteria over DIY meth-cookers was yet another convenient distortion in the War on Drugs that misrepresented the figures and disguised the real picture. The small-timers, what might be called the mom & pop labs—*I sold 3 grams and kept one for myself*—constituted the majority of those engaged in methedrine production, but they are in no way making most of the meth. The vast majority of meth labs in the United States—according to DEA statistics, 8,000 of the 8,300 seized in 2001—were home-user operations cook-ing no more that 280 hits at a time, and they represented only four percent of the total output. The bulk of the product—some estimates, published in various alternative newspapers, ran as high as 90 percent of all the meth consumed in the United States—was being manufactured elsewhere by much more organized and sinister operations. Law enforcement and the political drug warriors knew this, but preferred to divert attention from it. Chasing the DIY cookers could create a comfortable illusion that the War on Drugs was being won, while in fact it was being lost to the Mexican drug cartels. ●

ENTER THE AMEZCUA BROTHERS

WE REALLY ONLY KNOW ABOUT THE BROTHERS JESUS and Luis Amezcua Contreras because they were busted in 1998, and it took the Mexican authorities to bring them down despite the fact that the DEA called them the "leading distributors of methamphetamines in the United States," and Bill Clinton's Drug Czar, General Barry McCaffrey, described the Amezcuas as a "major threat to the US people." The Amezcuas' operation, however, set the pattern for the real manufacture of speed that, although the Amezcua Brothers remain in jail, possibly for the rest of their lives, continues relatively unchanged to this day. According to court records, the Amezcua Brothers, in the mid-1990s, imported an estimated 170 metric tons of ephedrine, made in India, China, Germany and the Czech Republic, in a single 18-month period, and processed it in their string of clandestine "superlabs," that were, with commercial-grade hardware, able to turn out 100,000 or even a million doses of good crystal meth in a two-day production run.

Some of these were in Mexico, across the southwest borders of the United States, but most were operating in the agribusiness open spaces of California's Central Valley, with its communities of migrant workers to provide natural cover. Easier by far, the Amezcuas reasoned— with the logic of Tony Montana in Brian De Palma's *Scarface*—to import truckloads of ephedrine across a border on the lookout for cocaine, heroin, and marijuana, than to attempt to mule over consignments of crystal meth. The superlabs of Amezcuas, and the other Mexican cartels whose names we don't know because they are still in business, were highly mobile. Equipment and chemicals were trucked in to some isolated property, set up quickly, then an intensive 48-hour production-run began. When the chemistry was complete, the entire lab was quickly torn down, the drugs went one way, and the equipment another. No fuss/no muss, and no time for authorities to get wind of what was going on. The superlabs only remained in place for two short days and then vanished, giving no time for law enforcement to pick up on noxious smells, suspicious comings and goings, detectable heat traces, or excess electricity usage—all of the signs that usually result in busts on more permanent operations.

By way of more cover, and also as a front for money laundering, the brothers had acquired more than 125 properties, including ranches, drug stores and travel agencies in the Mexican states of Jalisco and Colima, in Mexico City, and Baja California. Many of the drug stores were located in the border city of Tijuana, where according to the DEA, "they were used to facilitate the export of illegal methamphetamines and to help in the illegal import of ephedrine." The same drug stores may also have done a lucrative side business selling legitimate prescription drugs to the Americans who regularly stream across the border from San Diego to Tijuana looking for deals on the overpriced medications they could hardly afford to buy in the United States from unregulated and out of control pharmaceutical corporations. As far as can be gleaned from the official reports, the Amezcuas had, at the very least, a 10-year run as major speed suppliers. As early as 1993, Jesus and Luis Amezcua were indicted separately on drug charges in California, after a US Customs agent inadvertently discovered 3.4 metric tons of ephedrine on a plane traveling from Switzerland to Mexico. The consignment had come from a factory in India, and the Amezcuas' source was exposed. In the same year, Luis was also charged with murder.

Unfortunately, this was all done in their absence. They remained safe in Mexico, or if they did venture into the United States, they did it secretly, and no one was able to catch them. For three years, from 1995 to 1998, the United States government pressed for action by the Mexican authorities against the brothers, but it wasn't until 1998, after a federal grand jury in San Diego again indicted the Amezcua brothers on charges of manufacturing and distributing methamphetamine, and conspiracy to possess ephedrine, plus some related cocaine charges, that they were finally arrested by police in Mexico City. The Mexican courts, however, blocked extradition of the Amezcuas, frustrating the DEA who were already furious at the failure of earlier prosecutions. The extradition case against Luis Amezcua gained added notoriety when Mexican authorities balked at handing over a defendant in what could be a capital murder case, and in 2000, he was included on a White House list of suspected international drug kingpins subject to arrest, seizure, and a whole menu of financial penalties.

Ultimately, in 2004, the brothers were sentenced to long prison terms in Mexico. Jesus Amezcua, received fifty-three years and nine months and was ordered to pay a fine of $8,000 for trafficking in ephedrine. His brother, Luis was sentenced to 22 years and a fine of $6,500 on money-laundering charges. Prosecutors also unsuccessfully implicated the Amezcuas in the death of television comedian Francisco "Paco" Stanley, who was gunned down on a Mexico City freeway in 1999. Prosecutors alleged that Luis Amezcua ordered Stanley murdered because Stanley failed to pay off cocaine debts to the brothers, but Amezcua was acquitted of the charges, as were all the suspects charged in Stanley's killing. Despite the fact that the Amezcua brothers are in prison, United States authorities believe their organization still remains active.

The Amezcua brothers remain to this day the perfect model for a Mexican crystal meth cartel. For all we know they may still be running a version of their original operation from jail. Strange things happen in top-of-the-line drug cartels, as in the case of the legendary Colombian cocaine warlord Pablo Escobar who, when incarceration became inevitable, built himself his own luxury prison and ringed it with guards whose purpose was not to hold him inside, but to keep his enemies out. The Amezcua brothers were also the culmination of at least three decades of the Mexican underworld's desire for a piece of the lucrative American speed trade. Various Chicano gangs had, since the early days of street speed dealing in the 1960s, eyed the business with extreme covetousness. All attempts to carve themselves a slice had been thwarted by the Hells Angels and the other biker gangs, and later the neo-Nazis and white supremacists who had dedicated themselves both to maintaining a monopoly of the favorite trailer-park high, and seeing that its supply was a lily-white and ethnically exclusive profession.

Things might have stayed that way had not the DEA, looking for headlines, convictions, laudatory write-ups in national news magazines, formed an unwitting alliance with the Mexican mob. Again confirming that no room existed for either pragmatism or even common sense in the War on Drugs, US law enforcement broke the power and the lock on speed dealing enjoyed by the Hells bikers, but instead of cutting off all sources of crystal meth, which was supposedly their ultimate goal, they handed it to the more professional, more avaricious, and wholly more ruth-less Mexican underworld.

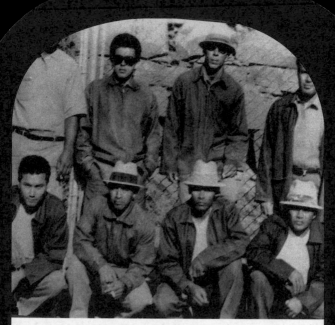

DON'T MESS WITH THE MEXICAN MAFIA

IN LOOSE talk and inaccurate news reports, the term "Mexican Mafia" is bandied around as though it was synonymous with all of organized crime in Mexico. Although it's easy to do, and sounds dramatic, it's something that is highly inaccurate and even dangerous. The Mexican Mafia is a precisely defined and highly exclusive organization, and certainly not a blanket term for any and every Chicano gangster. Also known as "La eMe" (Spanish for the letter "M"), the Mexican Mafia is one of the oldest prison gangs in the United States. Formed in the late 1950s by Chicano street gang members, mainly from a crew know as the Maravillas who were locked up in the Deuel Vocational Institution, a state prison in Tracy, California. The gang was founded by just 13 members, all from East Los Angeles, who initially referred to themselves as *Mexikanemi*—translated from Nahuatl as "He who walks with God in his heart."

As the power of the Mexican Mafia grew inside Deuel, the California Department of Corrections decided to break up the founding members by

transferring them to
other prison facilities, including San
Quentin. This move produced a completely opposite result to the one intended. Instead
of neutralizing "La eMe" inside the prison system, the Department of Corrections inadvertently
and unknowingly hosted a recruiting drive for new
members in prisons and juvenile correctional facilities that set the course for the Mexican Mafia as we
know it today, both in and out of the penal system.

The structure of the Mexican Mafia is almost totally copied from the popular concept of the Sicilian
Mafia in the United States—as we know it from the
Godfather movies and other pop-culture sources—
with a paramilitary structure, that includes generals,
captains, lieutenants and sergeants. Those ranking
below the sergeants are "soldiers," also called "carnales." Its major activities include extortion, drugs
(including a lucrative piece of the methamphetamine business) and contract murder. Not without
a certain irony, according to the FBI, La eMe has
been known to sub-contract for-hire killings to the
Aryan Brotherhood, the white supremacist prison
gang from whom, on the outside, they appropri-
ated the speed trade. The Mexican Mafia has a long
running alliance with the Aryan Brotherhood against
the Black Guerilla Family and other Afro-American
gangs, and also rival Latino gangs like rival group
Nuestra Familia. According to law enforcement, the
Mexican Mafia currently has no single overlord or
leader. Prison membership of the gang is believed to
consist of an elite numbering 150 or more who are
empowered to order killings, at least 1,000 associates—what would be called "made men" in the
Italian underworld—and close to 30,000 "carnales"
throughout the United States.

The Mexican Mafia made it to the movie
screen with in the 1992 movie *American Me*. The
film starred Edward James Olmos, who also copro-
duced and directed, as a character based on gang
leader Rodolfo Cadena. After the film's release,
Olmos allegedly received death threats, and
two consultants on the film were murdered.
Proving it's not healthy to mess with or
fictionalize the Mexican Mafia. ●

WITH NO PUN INTENDED, RECENT DEVELOPMENTS demonstrate that the Amezcua brothers may represent just the tiny tip of an enormous iceberg, and that the Mexican meth business has continued growing at a frightening rate since they were taken down. In 2006, Mexican authorities raided what they claimed was the largest methamphetamine lab anywhere in the Western Hemisphere in an industrial park in Guadalajara. The factory had 11 custom-designed pressure cookers capable of producing 400 pounds of crystal meth each day, which is about 20 times the production capacity of the Amezcuas' California labs in the 1990s. The DEA currently estimates that speed cartels transfer up $24 billion in hard cash from the United States to Mexico each year, and this hardly plausible sum was partially confirmed when, in 2007, Mexican authorities raided a mansion—described as a veritable fortress—in an exclusive and super up-market neighborhood in Mexico City that shared its location with the Israeli Embassy, the homes of some of the capital's wealthiest residents, and members of the international diplomatic corps.

A report in the *Los Angeles Times* on March 17, 2007 detailed how, "Authorities confiscated more than $200 million in US currency from methamphetamine producers in one of this city's ritziest neighborhoods, calling it the largest drug cash seizure in history. The seizure reflected the vast scope of an illegal drug trade linking Asia, Mexico and the United States, officials said. Two of the seven people arrested Thursday at a faux Mediterranean villa in the Lomas de Chapultepec neighborhood were Chinese nationals. The group was part of a larger drug-trafficking organization that imports 'precursor chemicals' from companies in India and China for processing into methamphetamine in Mexican 'super labs,' authorities said. The methamphetamine is eventually sold in the United States. The raid resulted from an investigation that began in December, when authorities seized 19 tons of pseudoephedrine, a cold medicine that is a key ingredient in the production of methamphetamine, at a Mexican port on the Pacific Coast. A legally registered Mexican company, listed by a trade association as the country's third-largest importer of pseudoephedrine, was implicated, officials said.

"Mexican drug-trafficking organizations have become increasingly important in the US methamphetamine trade, because the US has imposed tougher controls on the sale of the chemicals used to produce the highly addictive drug. President Felipe Calderon hailed the seizure as a major development in his government's war on drug traffickers, who have ravaged several Mexican cities and towns. 'We are working in a decisive manner to save our country and to keep Mexico safe and clean,' Calderon told an audience in Tijuana. 'I don't even want to imagine how many young people this gang poisoned with its drugs. But I can assure you, they will do it no longer.'

"Mexican officials said the cash seized was mostly in US $100 bills and weighed at least 4,500 pounds. Several machines for manufacturing pills were found at the site, but the group did not produce drugs there. The mansion appeared to serve as a financial operations center and cash storage facility." ●

CHAPTER 10

THE EPIDEMICS

"*TWEAKERS WHILE HIGH FIND IT HARD TO CONTROL their mouths, usually they click their tongues, move tongues around, their jaw moves, they bite their lips. Really hard-core tweakers pick at themselves—[marks that look like chicken-pox scabs are a telltale sign of hard use]. These people pick at themselves because they think the meth is coming out of their pores in the form of crystals and they try and pick the crystals out. Bad breath and dry mouth is another sure sign. Usually while tweaking the person's eyes are dilated, even in bright light.*"

—Anonymous

In the 2008 documentary film by Kevin Booth, *American Drug War: The Last White Hope*, Booth's camera crew returns from a ride-around with members of the Los Angeles Police Department to what looks like the central

Hollywood police station only to find a worse-for-wear, demented male speedfreak—he has the look of a damaged rock & roller in his early thirties who failed to ever find a band—actually sitting outside the station, smoking crystal meth in a pipe. The accompanying cops fall about laughing at this fool's mindless audacity, while the camera crew films his less than coherent comments. The vignette is funny, but also a bizarre confirmation of the awful stories that have circulated every two to three years since the 1990s of dangerous and debilitating methamphetamine epidemics in the American heartland.

Stories have been fed to the media, complete with TV footage at eleven, like that of the San Diego man in 1995, allegedly in the grip of amphetamine psychosis who managed to steal an Abrams tank (mercifully unarmed) from a local National Guard armory, and a rampage through suburban streets, crushing parked cars, and knocking over fire hydrants, and who was only stopped when police shot him dead as he moved his speeding juggernaut onto a stretch of freeway. The oblivious speedfreak in Hollywood and the San Diego madman in the tank represent two examples of extreme consumers at the end of the line that runs all the way back to the mansion in Mexico City with its $200 million in hundred dollar bills.

It would be pointless to deny that crystal meth is a problem, if for no other reason than it would appear to have brought drugs and the Drug War to suburban and rural America when it was previously concentrated in the major cities. If figures issued by the DEA are to be believed, meth use has grown by a multiple of five through the 1990s. In 1991 the DEA claimed to have seized some

21 million of what they call "dosage units" of methamphetamine throughout the United States. That number more than doubled to 48 million in 1992. In 1996 more than 74 million units were seized, and by 2002 the number rose to a scary 118 million hits of meth.

It is also pointless to pretend that teenagers using methamphetamine is anything but a very bad idea, especially bored teenagers with little education and few expectations of a purposeful or rewarding future. Beyond these statements, though, one can only wonder where cynicism ends and compassion starts in the Drug War. A lurid commercial by the Montana Meth Project starts with an elegantly lit photographic image of a filthy toilet in a down-market bar or club. The message reads: "NO ONE THINKS THEY'LL LOSE THEIR VIRGINITY HERE. METH WILL CHANGE THAT." Another image, in the same style, of an equally filthy prison cell delivers the message that "50% of Montana prison inmates are there due to meth."

The Montana Meth Project is a Montana-based anti-drug organization founded by the billionaire Thomas Siebel. Its major efforts are focused on developing advertising campaigns, primarily horror-heavy TV spots created by the San Francisco-based advertising agency Venables Bell & Partners, and billboards and back-up print materials designed to shock and awe viewers into realizing the dangers of methamphetamine use. The target audience is teenagers. The basic themes are amphetamine psychosis, and how speed is monstrously detrimental to users' health and living conditions. Other states, including Arizona, Idaho, and Illinois, have cloned the Montana project; it has been lauded by the George Bush White House and the DEA, and figures issued by the state claim a marked reduction in first time amphetamine use since the start of the project. On an official level it is hailed as a breakthrough success.

The shock tactics continue in the literature put out by the Montana Meth Project. One booklet states, "Long term methamphetamine abuse results in many damaging effects, including addiction. In addition to being addicted to methamphetamine, chronic methamphetamine abusers exhibit symptoms that can include violent behavior, anxiety, confusion, and insomnia. They also can display a number of psychotic features, including paranoia, auditory hallucinations, mood disturbances, and delusions (for example, the sensation of insects creeping on the skin, which is called "formication.") The paranoia can result in homicidal as well as suicidal thoughts. With chronic use, tolerance for methamphetamine can develop. In an effort to intensify the desired effects, users may take higher doses of the drug, take it more frequently, or change their method of drug intake. In some cases, abusers forego food and sleep while indulging in a form of binging known as a "run," injecting as much as a gram of the drug every 2 to 3 hours over several days until the user runs out of the drug or is too disorganized to continue. Chronic abuse can lead to psychotic behavior, characterized by intense paranoia, visual and auditory hallucinations, and out-of-control rages that can be coupled with extremely violent behavior."

On one hand, it's clear that the kids in Montana are not alright. On the other, the Montana Meth Project, now receiving state funds in addition to its original private financing, is a definite part of the War on Drugs, and echoes many of the drug warrior tactics we have already seen, that only ended badly when it became clear that the supposed cure was frequently ineffective, and worse than the disease. The same demonization of the user employed by Harry Anslinger, when he single-handedly started the Drug War back in the 1930s is one of Montana's weapons of choice. A Venables Bell & Partners commercial from the 2005/2006 season has a synopsis that reads: "In a shadowy drug den, a young boy tries methamphetamine for the first time. He is congratulated by dirty, drug-addicted people, who describe his future life as 'one of us.' One woman says that they will 'shoot up together,' two addicted men say that they and the boy will 'steal together…and we'll be sleepin' together, too.' The boy's protest that he is only trying it once is met with howls of laughter."

What we are really seeing is essentially a miniature vampire or zombie movie spiced with a very obvious dash of homophobia. All that seems to be missing is the killing and eating of neighborhood cats and kittens. The message is, in fact, not anti-drug, but anti–speedfreak. The difference is subtle, but also crucial. When used in the past, it has proved disastrous. Anslinger claimed that marijuana was a dangerous and addictive drug that inevitably turned those who used it, even just one time, into psychotic thrill killers. Potheads, doing their own research, quickly discovered that this was arrant nonsense, and now the Anslinger fantasy, as presented in the film *Reefer Madness*, is universally laughed at, and was even turned into a musical. The Venables Bell spot has a thicker layer of twenty-first century sophistication, but is similarly distorted. Casting the drug user as a universally alienating figure may well be the first mistake. There's nothing in which some teenagers take more delight than alienation. To abuse a drug that turns you into a bit player from *Night of the Living Dead* at least provides each new kid who turns to speed with an identity, and empowers a sense of leverage capable of shocking a world that prefers to deal with demographics rather than individuals.

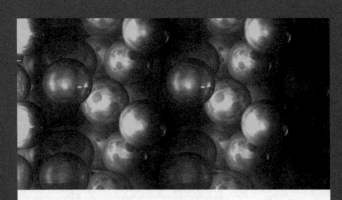

THE VIEW FROM THE OPPOSITE SIDE 1

"TRULY not giving a fuck is the only way to maintain perspective. In other words, there are worse things that can happen, than having to lay down and go to sleep for a week...no drug or state of mind is worth dying for, killing for, or doing hard time for...The American Speedfreak is not a lost soul. We know how to have fun between the first ether gasp and locking ourselves in the closet. A twisted wisdom creeps into those of us who manage to survive, a sort of collective uncon- sciousness, an unspoken Crankster ideology."

—Online poetry by a poet calling him or herself Speed Phreak on *Erowid.org*

THE ACCURACY OF MUCH OF THE MATERIAL THAT comes out of the Montana Meth Project is also questionable. The argument could be made that excess is justified if it warns the kids against the evils of drugs. Unfortunately, when the kids find out they've been misled, they tend to turn on the authority figures who misled them. They take the attitude—to borrow a line from the young Bob Dylan—"*propaganda all is phoney*." In the 1960s, the hippies were told that LSD 25 would turn your brain green and ultimately destroy it, which only seemed to make the psychedelic generation more anxious to trip. Is there, for instance, really such a phenomenon as "formication"? Certainly speedfreaks tend to scratch themselves. Dehydration from speed and toxins in the drug make this a given, but whether they come complete with full blown insect hallucinations is entirely another matter. The hallucinations may well come from the imagination of one impressionable teen telling caseworkers what they want to hear, while he or she is caught up in a media-driven moral panic, because moral panic is what's essentially being created. The term "moral panic" was coined by sociologist Stanley Cohen, the Martin White Professor of Sociology at the London School of Economics, in his 1972 study *Folk Devils and Moral Panics* in which he defines it as "the reaction by a group of people based on the false or exaggerated perception that some cultural behavior or group, frequently a minority group or a subculture, is dangerously deviant and poses a menace to society." According to Cohen, the tools for creating moral panics include "emotive language

163

and images such as monsters, decay and crisis to empha-size the acuteness of the problem. Medical language can also be used out of context such as the word 'epidemic.' Statistics are often misused or written in such a way that makes the reader think the problem is worse than it is; for example, '400% greater' will make most think that some-thing is 400 times higher rather than 4 times." The most telling of his observations concerns the demonization of a group: "Sometimes the chosen group does not even exist and those that do are mostly socially or economically mar-ginal. Often the media can portray a group in ways that don't really exist and the group will eventually live up to the stereotype created for them."

Although it must be stressed that, while far too many Montana teens may in reality be having real problems with speed, the ultimate value of the shock tactics of the Meth Project have to be held in question, perhaps for no other reason than many Montana speedfreaks took their first hit of speed in a context that was totally sanctioned by parents, physicians, teachers, and the law. This first taste wasn't manufactured in some Mexican superlab, or even a home cooker in a trailer park. It was created by a totally respectable pharmaceutical corporation and came in the form of one of two drugs—either Ritalin or Adderall.

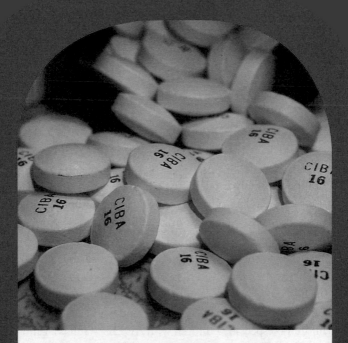

THE VIEW FROM THE OPPOSITE SIDE 2

"FROM my experience both drugs produce a calming sensation like a strong nicotine buzz. Like marijuana both make you zoned out. Adderall seems to do this the best, more so than Ritalin. The reason for the feeling of being zoned out is because they block the signals of thoughts in the brain, leaving you with a calm feeling. It clears the mind so that you can think of only one thing at a time. Adderall can be euphoric especially when it first begins to kick in. This usually lasts for a half and hour. Ritalin has a stronger euphoric feeling especially with the extended release version called Concerta, which actually works to calm you down by increasing the dopamine in the brain. The euphoric feeling of Ritalin lasts about an hour and the speedy awakeness feelings usually last for three. When either of these drugs are taken in large quantities like 150 mg of Adderall or Ritalin, the effects can last all day."

—Notes published online on the recreational use of Ritalin and Adderall by a character using the name Mad Scientist

RITALIN IS THE TRADE NAME FOR THE CHEMICAL compound methylphenidate, a drug with a molecular structure that has what is known as an "amphetamine backbone," and so creates similar effects to that of amphetamine and methamphetamine. Despite this, it is chiefly prescribed to children for attention deficit disorder (ADD), and attention deficit and hyperactivity disorder (ADHD). The odd paradox with Ritalin is that, when used by adults, it acts more like a variation of any kind of speed, but with children—especially children with ADHD—it has a calming effect, allowing them to focus their attention. It has accordingly, since the 1960s, been prescribed to children as a form of tranquilizer, and in such quantities that it has been seen as a means of child management, rather than medication for any specific problem.

In 1996, the United Nations reported that 10 to 12 percent of all male schoolchildren in the United States were taking Ritalin, although only approximately three to five percent of the population has either ADD or ADHD. Unconfirmed but quite plausible stories still circulate that Columbine high school shooter Eric Harris was a Ritalin child, as were 15-year-old Shawn Cooper of Notus, Idaho, and 15-year-old T.J. Soloman of Conyers, Georgia when they opened fire at their schools, while the Oregon teenager Kip Kinkel was prescribed both Ritalin and Prozac when he murdered both his parents, and then opened fire in his school cafeteria later the same day, killing two and wounding 22. A new picture has started to emerge of kids on Ritalin as baleful time-bomb zombies,

with maliciously narcissistic parents who are only interested in keeping them quiet, and doctors who have been
totally corrupted by the pharmaceutical industry. At the
dysfunctional extreme, tales have even spread of parents
taking their children's Ritalin. This may of course be as
much of a possible exaggeration as the Montana Meth
Projects demonization of methamphetamine and speedfreaks, but it all provides an uncomfortable parallel to the
usual patterns of speedfreak behavior.

Adderall has, in recent years, become a rival to Ritalin in the treatment of ADD and ADHD, especially
among children and adolescents. While Ritalin had only
a molecular "amphetamine spine," Adderall is described
by its maker, Shire Pharmaceuticals, as "a pharmaceutical
psychostimulant composed of mixed amphetamine salts."
Adderall is prescribed in pill form, and also time-release
capsules that are sold as Adderall XR. Although Adderall
has not been around as long as Ritalin, and consequently
not amassed the same shroud of doubt regarding the ad-
visability of its use, it has already run into problems. Early
in 2005, Health Canada, the Canadian government's national health care provider, suspended all sales of Adderall
XR after data collected by Shire Pharmaceuticals suggested
there was a link between the drug and the sudden deaths
of a dozen American children who were prescribed the
drug. As research went further, it suggested that the use
of Adderall resulted, at an early age, in an increased risk of
cardiac defect. In the United States, however, the fact that
more than 37 million prescriptions for Adderall were filled
between 2000 and 2004 was cited as a reason for the US
Food and Drug Administration to do nothing. Siding with

the manufacturer, the FDA claimed that it could find no increased risk of sudden death among Adderall XR users beyond the normal rate for the general population, and so no action was needed.

And so the paradox stands as just one more contradiction in the War On Drugs. On one hand, a massive advertising campaign, instituted in Montana and backed by both the DEA and the White House, attempts to sell the concept of meth-monster amphetamine addiction, while the state also jails a large percentage of its local speedfreaks. On the other, the FDA approves the use of a prescribed amphetamine as "a pharmaceutical psycho-stimulant" for children. The phrase "go figure" seems hardly expansive enough to express how perplexing the behavior of our drug warriors has become, and yet, what else can be said? ●

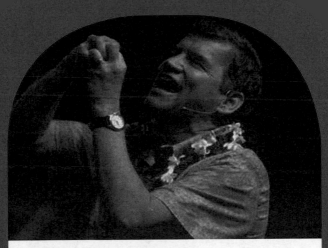

METH IN THE MEGACHURCH

COLORADO SPRINGS, Colorado (CNN November 4th, 2006)—The Rev. Ted Haggard agreed Saturday to resign as leader of the megachurch he started in his basement more than 20 years ago after its independent investigative board said he was guilty of "sexually immoral conduct."

On Friday, Haggard admitted he had received a massage from a Denver man who claimed the prominent pastor had paid him for sex over three years. Haggard also admitted he had bought methamphetamine.

Haggard, in an interview with CNN affiliate KUSA, denied having sex with Mike Jones and said he did not use the drug and threw it away.

After the allegations were made public, Haggard resigned as president of the influential National Association of Evangelicals, an umbrella group representing more than 45,000 churches with 30 million members.

He also temporarily stepped aside as pastor of the 14,000-member New Life Church.

But on Saturday overseers of the church recommended he be permanently removed.

"We, the Overseer Board of New Life Church, have concluded our deliberations concerning the moral failings of Pastor Ted Haggard," a statement from the church said. ●

THE THIRD WORLD ALTERNATIVE

THE 2001 RIDLEY SCOTT MOVIE *BLACK HAWK DOWN*, tells the story of a mission in Somalia on October 3, 1993, during which nearly 100 US Army Rangers, commanded by Capt. Mike Steele, were dropped by helicopter deep into the capital city of Mogadishu to capture two top lieutenants of a Somali warlord. Miscalculations on the part of the Rangers turned a simple capture and extraction into a massive firefight between US troops and hundreds of Somali gunmen, and resulted in the downing of two US Black Hawk helicopters in Mogadishu. More casualties were sustained as other detachments of Rangers attempted to rescue their comrades. During the course of the movie, reference is made to a drug called khat (pronounced "kot") that supposedly kept the Somali warlords' machine-gun and RPG militias fighting

171

crazy. At the time, Tom Brokaw had reported on *NBC Nightly News* how "Somali thugs high on khat" were patrolling the streets of Mogadishu.

The temptation might be to dismiss khat as some rudimentary herbal version of amphetamine from the horn of Africa and parts of the Middle East. A little research reveals that Khat is the product of the young leaves of a flowering evergreen shrub some six to 12 feet tall native to east Africa and southern Arabia know as *Catha edulis*, and, traditionally, the chewing of khat or infusing the leaves in hot water to make a drink predates the use of coffee and is consumed in similar social contexts. Further digging reveals that the use of khat has possibly been used for close to 3,000 years, dating back to the ancient Egyptians who considered the leaves a "divine food" which could produce a transcendental state called "apotheosis" in which a user became god-like.

For centuries after that, khat was chewed in moderation, to alleviate fatigue and reduce appetite. Over use, however, was reported to produce delusions, paranoia, and hallucinations. All in all, the effects of khat sounded a lot like those of amphetamine. The British explorer Sir Richard Burton mentions the use and effects of khat in his book *First Footsteps in East Africa* (1856) and tells how the leaf was introduced to Yemen from Ethiopia somewhere between the thirteenth and fifteen centuries, and also reveals that its medicinal use is mentioned in the New Testament. The assumption remained that khat was a third-world curio, only used in the West by seekers after more exotic highs, or was brought in for use by emigrants from the source countries as an herbal reminder of home.

In 1854, the Malay writer Abdullah bin Abdul Kadir noted that the custom of chewing Khat was prevalent in Al Hudaydah in Yemen: "I observed a new peculiarity in this city—everyone chewed leaves as goats chew the cud. There is a type of leaf, rather wide and about two fingers in length, which is widely sold, as people would consume these leaves just as they are; unlike betel leaves, which need certain condiments to go with them, these leaves were just stuffed fully into the mouth and munched. Thus when people gathered around, the remnants from these leaves would pile up in front of them. When they spat, their saliva was green. I then queried them on this matter: 'What benefits are there to be gained from eating these leaves'? To which they replied, 'None whatsoever, it's just another expense for us as we've grown accustomed to it'. Those who consume these leaves have to eat lots of ghee and honey, for they would fall ill otherwise. The leaves are known as Kad."

Khat has this long historical record, but very little evidence seemed to point to it playing any significant role in the modern American or European drug scenes except that it might somehow be connected to a drug named "cat," a variation on speed that seemed largely mythic and anecdotal. Thus to learn from a November 2006 story by Sean Gardiner in the *Village Voice* that "over the past year khat was second only to marijuana in total pounds seized by US Customs agents nationwide— more than double that of cocaine, and 28 times more than methamphetamine"—came as something of a surprise. Surprise was magnified when Gardiner continued. "Just this past summer, authorities busted the first substantial khat-trafficking ring in the United States. Operation Somali Express resulted in 44 men and women arrested in connection with [the] importing of 25 tons of khat the previous 18 months, with an estimated street value of $10 million. The head of New York's FBI office then expressed concern that khat profits were being used to fund terrorists associated with Al Qaeda."

Shortly before Sean Gardiner wrote his khat story—the gist of which was that, as far as Gardiner could see, khat was being used primarily by Somali immigrants and others from the same region, and that it was impossible to find in New York City, and certainly did not seem to have penetrated the New York drug culture—a khat segment appeared on ABC TV's *Nightline*, and a DEA agent claimed khat was being "marketed in all cross-sections of our country." The show ended with a note of ominous drama. "Today's raid is the nation's first attempt to stop this new drug before it's able to take hold. The question is, will it work"?

More reports of khat busts followed. Over 700 pounds of khat in railroad containers was seized by Philadelphia police officers in September of 2007, and in December of the same year, federal authorities seized more than 400 pounds of khat at the Salt Lake City airport. Deputies arrested two men from Utah, Patrick Bahati and Sherif Kadir Sirage, for attempting to import a combined 450 pounds from Ethiopia. Officials say the two tried to pass the khat off as various spices for personal use. If convicted, they could face up to 20 years.

To discover what the uproar was all about, and why authorities seemed so bent out of shape about the dangers of khat needed a cross reference to the work of Dr.

Richard Glennon, Professor of Medicinal Chemistry at the Medical College of Virginia, who began studying the molecular structure of *Catha edulis* in the 1980s. From information culled from multiple sources it appears that through his research Glennon found that cathinone, the active chemical in the plant, is structurally similar to amphetamine. He made changes to the molecule to make it more active than cathinone. "We gave it the name, methcathinone." He continues with what seems a strange pride: "Methcathinone is to cathinone what methamphetamine, or speed, is to amphetamine. Methcathinone is 10 times more potent than cocaine." The even stranger part of the story is that is that Glennon takes even more pride in the fact that he worked with the DEA, providing the agency with data on the effects of methcathinone on possible users in order that they could classify methcathinone as dangerous in 1993.

He appears to be saying that he perfected a process to create a new and potentially dangerous drug, but then blew the whistle on it himself to prevent a possible methcathinone "epidemic," similar to the ones caused by methamphetamine. The problem starts when Glennon goes on to claim that, because of his work, the DEA shut down, "more than 50 cat labs in the past few years." One has to ask how, if methcathinone was Glennon's unique discovery and he immediately passed the information on to the DEA, where did these illegal cat labs, that were presumably processing *Catha edulis* into methcathinone, get the recipe? Glennon's reported response proves a little contradictory, since as soon as he published his work on *Catha edulis* and methcathinone, a Russian scientist contacted him and said that methcathinone was "a widely abused drug in the former Soviet Union, second only to alcohol."

At this point, the story starts to become even more confused. Glennon seems to claim that, "a Midwestern ex-university student" figured out in the early 1990s how to make the drug, and this individual's "discovery" spawned methcathinone or "cat" laboratories throughout Michigan, Illinois, and Wisconsin, and "inhaling, swallowing and shooting up cat created a major drug problem in that region." The drug known as "cat" certainly circulated, especially among American speedfreaks, but hardly ever rose to the level of a "major drug problem." An anonymous commentator on *erowid.org* comes close to being patronizingly dismissive of cat:

"On the brighter side, this is not a drug I've written off. In reasonable dosages, it's an effective mood elevator producing a very extroverted high, doesn't induce "motor mouth," a real party drug... sorta makes you wanna dance. It never threatens to take you down that mission-from-God, don't-bother-me, I-can't-stop-now road that comes from believing your own bullshit on a speed run. It goes great with beer, less saturated fat than pretzels! I guess that about covers it as far as how a CAT plucks MY wires, remember though, in all likelihood I've burned over a lot more of these circuits than you, a less trodden synaptic superhighway may invoke entirely different responses, for better or worse. I have found it impossible to include a recommended first dosage in good conscience...please be careful, and reference other literature for this."

All street indications would seem to follow the one above and define cat as never being more than a minor luminary in the amphetamine pantheon, and certainly not some new monster amphetamine that's "10 times more potent than cocaine." If cat is so small time, why did the DEA make such a major fuss about it? And where were all those bales of *Catha edulis* leaves going and to what purpose? In his *Village Voice* story Sean Gardiner seemed equally surprised. "My search for khat began late in September after the Queens district attorney sent out a press release detailing an arrest for khat possession. In 15 years covering crime, I had never heard of the substance. Apparently, after picking up a 13-pound box of khat, workers at a Queens UPS warehouse tipped off police. As the cops moved in for the pinch, the suspects were still sitting in their car outside UPS contentedly munching mouthfuls of the leaves. The press release went on to surprise me with the news that khat 'is in the same legal category as heroin or cocaine.'"

All in all, this hardly sounds like a mass drug interdiction. This was no 25 tons of khat worth $10 million. Much more like a bunch of Somalis picking up a box of homeland high, unaware of the penalties involved. The cat story seems to gather more and more anomalies as it progresses. Tales surface that cat was not in fact created by "a Midwestern ex-university student," but introduced to this country by "a man of Russian descent" who "may have received the recipe from his relatives in the former Soviet Union." So who is this man, an outlaw chemist, part of the Russian mob? This single nugget of information seems to be all that anyone has written. Every trail to the true origin of cat seems to tail off into more unanswered questions, the major one being, if the DEA believes there is such a thing as a major cat epidemic, where are all the desperate cat users? Individuals who have used the drug sometime/ onetime are easily located, but regular users are impossible to find? The meth smoker can babble to a camera crew right outside the Hollywood police station, and tweakers roam the streets of towns and cities all over this land, but the catheads are apparently so deep underground that they take on an air of fiction?

The posts on online drug culture messages boards reflect a similar confusion. As in, "My question is if anyone knows anything about methacathinone (sp?) aka CAT. A friend of mine cooked some up using pseudoephedrine as a base. I was told that it's really bad for you (more than your common amphetamine) and was really adamant that I never try it again. I found it to be more subtle than meth and had none of the crash when it was over. It had a pleasant buzz and kept you going. Does anyone have any experience with this drug?"

No one volunteered any further information, and ignorance of cat seemed so all consuming that none of the usual know-it-all, self-appointed, online pundits bothered to point out that, if the friend cooked up cat from pseudoephedrine rather than cathinone, the active chemical in khat leaves, the friend wasn't cooking cat at all, but some home-made variant of methamphetamine. This may well be a clue to the real truth, and a lot less strange than fiction. The suggestion would appear to be, if you have managed to cook up some form of highly dubious speed—perhaps by the Nazi method—that no customer or friend would accept as crystal meth, simply call it cat and hope that the consumers don't figure out what's been pulled on them.

Another alternative to consider is that the tons of khat netted in the Operation Somali Express, plus the 700 pounds of leaves seized in Philadelphia, and the 400 pounds at Salt Lake City airport were loads of precursor intended for a large-scale cat production run, but we were saved from a khat epidemic by the efforts of the DEA and local law, and the nation should be grateful for their unswerving vigilance that saved us from the horror of a new and powerful drug. An equally plausible explanation is that the DEA, FBI, and Customs Services intentionally promoted Dr. Glennon's exaggerated data with their own overstated claims of khat seizures in order to increase fears of an impending khat epidemic. When the epidemic failed to materialize, the drug warriors in the three agencies could take credit for thwarting a potential horror. In other words, with the exception of some small and seemingly elusive supplies, cat—in any kind of mass distribution—was largely the figment of a conspired propaganda campaign designed to court public approval and increase drug warrior funding.

A guitar player from England tells the story about how, to supplement his lamentable lack of a musical income, he went in on a deal with a group of stoners to import khat leaves under the guise of herbal products. The idea was to import the Somali habit of chewing the leaves for a mild speed rush, introduce it as a legal drug-culture novelty, and make a substantial profit in the process. In the UK, Khat is not a controlled substance, and recent attempts to reclassify it had been rejected, so the scheme was in no way criminal. It failed because it was simply too strange. The majority of Brit speedfreaks and potheads weren't ready to walk around with a Somali-style wad of leaves stuffed in their cheek. The enterprise was little short of disaster, and strapped for cash, the wanna-be khat cartel began chewing their own merchandise. How was that? The guitar player looked embarrassed and shook his head. It had been mildly distracting, weird and quietly jagged, and after prolonged use they had all felt unfocused and ill. These Englishmen lacked a Somali's cultural and chemical tolerance for khat. When asked if he and his partners had considered cooking the cathinone into methcathinone, the guitar player nodded. They thought of it, but hardly deemed themselves cat-cooking material. Breaking the leaves down into cathinone made it a Class C drug and [that would have] crossed the line into criminality. "And anyway, we were hardly the kind of people to be fucking with explosive and corrosive chemicals." ●

THE PORNOGRAPHY OF INFORMATION

"*MANIACS GENERALLY DO NOT HAVE TOO MUCH BE-tween the ears. They can pick up a book and they don't get past the table of contents.*"   —Steve Preisler/Uncle Fester

"*You need to be able to read ideas that any right-thinking person would vehemently oppose, and YOU need to figure out if YOU should oppose these ideas, embrace them, or ignore them. It should be up to YOU to decide what you believe in, not someone warming a chair in Washington, D.C.*"
          —Jeff Hunter, Temple of the Screaming Electron

Uncle Fester is a character who just lives to fuck with explosive and corrosive chemicals. In cartoon, film, and TV series, Fester is the demented bald uncle with the weird eyes from *The Addams Family*. In the underground world of subversive publishing, he provides a pen name for an industrial chemist named Steve Preisler. Preisler, who lives as single father with his two children in a middle-class, residential neighborhood of Green Bay, Wisconsin, works by day in an electroplating factory he's dubbed "the rat hole," but at night, like some bizarre comic book superhero he assumes his alter ego and writes what many in authority consider some of the most threatening books in print today. One example of his work is *Home Workshop Explosives*—a fairly self-explanatory title, although, in a review, David Harber, author of *Guerrilla's Arsenal*, did note that "although the chemistry is solid," the chapter on Detonation Systems "borders on insanity." Fester is also the author of *Vest Busters* that details easy methods for creating Teflon-coated bullets, and other body-armor penetrating ammunition. His *Silent Death* describes how to manufacture nerve gases and poisons, and *Bloody Brazilian Knife Fightin' Techniques* is again self-explanatory. In this context, however, Uncle Fester's first book, *Secrets of Methamphetamine Manufacture* and the much later follow-up *Advanced Techniques of Clandestine Psychedelic & Amphetamine Manufacture*, are the most relevant.

Secrets of Methamphetamine Manufacture, published by Loompanics and now in its seventh edition, offers a detailed guide to the making of crystal methamphetamine six different ways, plus recipes for synthesizing MDMA or MDA, and Methcathinone from ephedrine. It also contains syntheses for precursor materials including ephedrine and the original Hells Angels favorite phenylacetone or P2P. As such, it has been a constant irritant to the drug warriors since it first came out in the early 1980s. On a deeper level, the cat and mouse, Drug War circumstances that caused Preisler to write the book in the first place provided yet another example of the inroads the drug warriors feel free to make into some of our most cherished freedoms.

Having graduated from Marquette University with chemistry & biology degrees, Preisler found himself, in 1983, arrested for methamphetamine possession and given probation. A year later he was busted again for meth, and tossed in the Waupun Correctional Institution. The initial charges were only for a few grams of meth, but then the DEA brought back credit card bills that allegedly showed Uncle Fester had been buying large quantities of ephedrine, which, prosecutors charged, was proof of intent to manufacture. Fester's revenge on a system he had come to loath was, while still in jail, to start writing the most subversive material he could imagine—and what could be more subversive than how-to books on drugs and explosives. Writing on his own website, Fester is clearly pleased with what he has achieved:

"Since 1985, everybody's favorite Uncle has been writing the books which have defined the field of clandestine chemistry. My books have been described as the pinnacle of 20th century underground writing, and through them I have transformed this genre. Prior to my typewriter driven blitzkrieg, underground books were generally entertaining, but sorely lacking in technical prowess and veracity. Your Uncle has retained the entertaining qualities of the classic underground press while presenting accurate and reliable information in the clearest manner I can muster."

Law enforcement, the media, and federal and local authorities, on the other hand, definitely don't think of

Fester as their favorite Uncle. They have more than once dubbed him "The Most Dangerous Man in America." They fail to see his work as being simply in the tradition all anarchic and subversive agitprop, and reject his statement that he just enjoys, "the thrill of writing a book that skirts the edge and then maybe beyond, a book that offends." Instead, the powers-that-be claim Preisler is deliberately supplying drug dealers and terrorists with crucial information. In support of this claim, they alleged that members of the Japanese Aum Shinrikyo cult, who killed 12 people in 1995 by releasing Sarin nerve gas in the Tokyo subway system, had Fester's *Silent Death*, with its chapter on Sarin, among their research materials. A less than repentant Preisler told the CBS news show *48 Hours* that he was "rather sad that that happened but I don't feel responsibility for what they did. They're the ones who did it." Though, in another interview, Uncle Fester castigated the Aum cultists for their sloppy workmanship.

If, however, the US government v Uncle Fester had remained a war of words, that might have been acceptable, but in March of 2001 police in Denver, Colorado decided that they would make a move to prevent Fester's books from being sold or even read by the American people. This was the day that Denver cops raided the trailer of a suspected meth cooker, and while searching place, found Fester's *Secrets of Methamphetamine Manufacture,* and *Advanced Techniques of Clandestine Psychedelic Drug Laboratories*, plus a receipt from a bookstore called the Tattered Cover. The following day two detectives showed up at the bookstore with a search warrant. The officers claimed the buyer's identity was critical to their case. The store refused under the First Amendment to give out any such information, which set the stage for a landmark court battle.

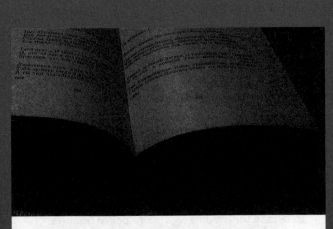

WHEN AN INDIVIDUAL'S RIGHT TO PRIVACY COLLIDES WITH THE PURSUIT OF LAW ENFORCEMENT, WHAT SHOULD YIELD?

THAT QUESTION was the centerpiece of a unique panel at the Denver Press Club December 12, where discussion focused on a controversial case involving a suspected criminal's alleged purchase of drug cookbooks from the Tattered Cover bookstore in Denver. The case has generated national attention, and is expected to land in the Colorado Supreme Court sometime next year—and perhaps even the US Supreme Court. The facts of the case are as follows: In March, police in suburban Denver

busted a methamphet-
amine lab in a mobile home. Within
the mobile home, the police found two
books: *The Construction and Operation of Clandestine Drug Laboratories* by "Jack B. Nimble" and
*Advanced Techniques of Clandestine Psychedelic
and Amphetamine Manufacture* by "Uncle Fester."
Outside in the trash the cops found a shipping
envelope containing an invoice number from the
Tattered Cover.

Believing that the invoice number was connected to the purchase of the books, and therefore
would lead to a key suspect among several people
who inhabited the mobile home, the police were
granted a search warrant to track down the invoice
at the Tattered Cover. Bookstore owner Joyce Meskis refused to cooperate, saying that protecting her
customers' privacy is paramount. Speaking to an
audience of about 40 people, the panel at the press
club included Meskis, her attorney, law enforcement personnel involved in the case, a local judge,
and a representative of the Privacy Foundation,
which cosponsored the event spearheaded by the
Colorado Bar Association.

Meskis told the gathering that she refused
to release the invoice records to police because
it would set a disturbing precedent that she felt
would violate First Amendment rights. Police
countered that the invoice was a key piece of
evidence to track down the purchaser of the drug
cookbooks, and would help them pursue their
criminal case. Most on the panel agreed that there
need to be crystal clear guidelines for the police
to obtain search warrants, particularly when the
evidence sought relates to reading material. A
member of the audience said she supported the
right of bookstores and vendors on the Internet to
sell and distribute provocative materials, without
fear of action by law enforcement.

—*Justin Rickard writing for the Privacy Foundation.*

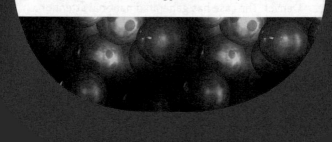

INITIALLY A COLORADO COURT RULED IN FAVOR OF the police request and against the Tattered Cover, a decision that the store's owner, Joyce Meskis challenged in the Colorado Supreme Court, making clear to the media that, "It's not our job to do the police's work for them." Fortunately the Colorado Supreme Court ultimately overturned the previous judge's ruling on the matter, handing down a unanimous six-zero decision in the bookstore's favor. For the moment, the efforts of law enforcement to stem the free passage of information and dump First Amendment rights in their supposed priority of freeing the nation from the scourge of drugs had been thwarted, and in Colorado at least, the principle that information and its free circulation—any information and any circulation—was unassailable had been upheld.

Among those who should have been heartened by this decision are Jeff Hunter and J.C. Stanton, who run the website *totse.com* also know as the Temple of the Screaming Electron, which carries multiple postings on many "subversive resources"—outlaw drug production, home bomb making, locksmithing, rocket launchers, religion, erotica, and something called "the conspiracy of ugly and stupid people." The "Nazi method" of meth cooking reproduced earlier comes from an anonymous post on *totse.com*, and the vast majority of the articles on the site are contributed by reader/writers whose numbers run into the hundreds of thousands if not millions. Hunter confirms the traffic on the site's FAQ page. "In January 2007 *totse.com* averaged 3.6 million hits per day, and each month the daily average goes up by a few hundred thousand hits," and all of these visitors pass this disclaimer: NOTICE: TO ALL CONCERNED Certain text files and messages contained on this site deal with activities and devices which would be in violation of various federal, state, and local laws if actually carried out or constructed. The webmasters of this site do not advocate the breaking of any law. Our text files and message bases are for informational purposes only. We recommend that you contact your local law enforcement officials before undertaking any project based upon any information obtained from this or any other web site. We do not guarantee that any of the information contained on this system is correct, workable, or factual. We are not responsible for, nor do we assume any liability for, damages resulting from the use of any information on this site.

Another writer who, like Uncle Fester, found himself in law enforcement's crosshairs because of a book he had published, and the details it went into regarding illegal drugs and their manufacture was no less than Dr. Alexander Shulgin. In his own field Dr. Shulgin is a revered figure. A summation of his work in a *New York Times* profile reads, "For 40 years, working in plain sight of the law and publishing his results, Shulgin has been a one-man psychopharmacological research sector. (Timothy Leary called him one of the century's most important scientists.) By Shulgin's own count, he has created nearly 200 psychedelic compounds." Shulgin has already been mentioned in this book as researcher who resurrected MDMA (Ecstasy) as a psycho-therapeutic in 1967, and then, nine years later, develop a new method of synthesis, and introduced

MDMA to Oakland psychologist Leo Zeff, who used the drug as an aid to talk therapy.

In 1991, Dr. Shulgin and his wife Ann wrote a book entitled *PiHKAL* about psychedelic phenethylamines (full title *Phenethylamines I Have Known and Loved: A Chemical Love Story*.) The book comes in two parts. The first is the couples fictionalized autobiography, the second contains detailed synthesis instructions for over 200 psychedelic compounds, most of which Shulgin personally invented. One of the Shulgin's major reasons for writing *PiHKAL* was to ensure that the details of his discoveries would not be confined to professional research labs and find their way to the general public, because Shulgin devoutly believes, despite all government propaganda to the contrary, that psychedelic drugs are invaluable tools for self-exploration. The recipe for synthesizing MDMA in PiHKAL remains one of the most common clandestine methods of manufacture.

Unfortunately, in 1994, two years after the publication of *PiHKAL*, the DEA raided Shulgin's lab. Agents claimed there were problems with his record keeping, and stripped Shulgin of his Schedule 1 license which allowed him to work with otherwise illegal substances. He was further fined $25,000 for the possession of anonymous samples sent to him for testing. The reason for the raid was clearly the information revealed in *PiHKAL*, and this was confirmed by Richard Meyer, the spokesman for DEA's San Francisco Field Division. "It is our opinion that those books are pretty much cookbooks on how to make illegal drugs. Agents tell me that in clandestine labs that they have raided, they have found copies of those books." What

Meyer failed to mention was that Shulgin had sold over 40,000 copies of *PiHKAL*, and that the book could, in theory, show up just about anywhere.

In 1997, the Shulgins wrote a second book, *TiHKAL* (*Tryptamines I Have Known and Loved: The Continuation*). Like its predecessor, it is in two parts; a fictionalized autobiography, continuing where *PiHKAL* left off, and then a collection of essays that explore everything from psychotherapy and the Jungian mind, to DMT in nature, ayahuasca, and the War on Drugs plus a detailed synthesis manual for 55 more psychedelics. So far, the DEA has not made a move.

Writers like Alexander Shulgin, Uncle Fester, and websites like *totse.com* and the more exclusively drug-oriented, *erowid.org*, (also known as The Vault of Erowid) represent a front line in the defense of genuine freedom of speech. Without them, the only information on recreational drugs permitted to the American people would be the slanted propaganda dispensed by everyone from Harry Anslinger to The Montana Meth Project. If the drug warriors had their way, they would ignore the Constitution, trash The Bill of Rights, and do away with the provisions for free expression in The First Amendment. Their mission is to close what H. G. Wells called the "doors in the wall," the same doors quoted and opened by Aldous Huxley.

Crucial information would be filtered and censored like a form of pornography, and the people who have already crafted arbitrary, unworkable, and arguably immoral laws to govern which chemicals we may put in our bodies would have the equally arbitrary power to dictate what we can write or read, talk about, or ultimately even think. Too many of our leaders, past and present, have been infected with the idea that they were elected to be obeyed. The sooner they are disabused of that megalomaniacal notion the better off the nation's mental health will become.

For all practical purposes, and allowing for the reality that, despite their best efforts and the fortunes in taxpayer money spent by the drug warriors, millions of us still really make our own decisions as to which drugs we want to take and which ones we want to leave alone. Wanna smoke a joint, do a line of speed, drop some acid, or throw back a shot of Jack Daniels? If so asked, very few respond negatively simply because to do so would be illegal, the president wouldn't like it, or because they heard that drug money supports terrorism. We don't follow absurd advice of Nancy Reagan and "just say no" like mindless sheep. Many more Americans than one might imagine still tend to make up their own minds, if they're given all the relevant facts and contents, and are not kept on a diet of self-serving corporate/government disinformation. Many Americans—certainly a large minority, if not the majority—also feel they have been lied to so often that they no longer take the pronouncements coming out of Washington, the Statehouse, or the mayor's office at face value.

Free people are not, almost by definition, obedient people. They tend to question. They want to know why. If those in power create an information vacuum around a specific subject like drug use, people like Alexander Shulgin and Uncle Fester, each in his different way, is acting out of a unique form of patriotism. Okay, so Uncle Fester appears to many as an angry renegade, but this country has a long and proud tradition of angry renegades who

191

annoy, who puncture bubbles, and who expose what the authoritarians in power would rather keep hidden, and what makes them uncomfortable. The unfettered truth-teller is essential if we are to maintain the freedom of a free society. We may not like the subjects he chooses to tell the truth about, but as long as he continues to challenge the forces that might want to put a muzzle on him, we can be assured the information we need to make fully informed choices, to protect ourselves, and council our children, is still moving freely. ●

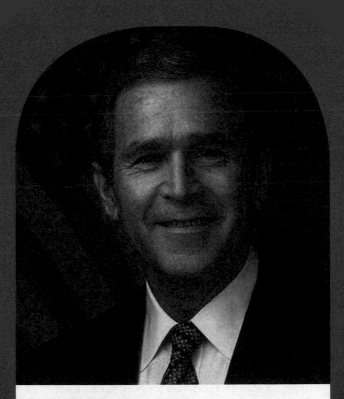

∩ATIONAL
METHAMPHETAMINE
AWARENE∫∫ DAY, 2006

A Proclamation by the President of the
United States of America

METHAMPHETAMINE abuse shatters families
and threatens our communities. On National
Methamphetamine Awareness Day, we underscore
the dangers of methamphetamine and reaffirm
our collective responsibility to combat all forms
of drug abuse.

Methamphetamine is a powerfully addictive
drug that dramatically affects users' minds and
bodies. Chronic use can lead to violent behavior,
paranoia, and an inability to cope with the ordinary
demands of life. Methamphetamine abusers can
transform homes into places of danger and de-
spair by neglecting or endangering the lives of
their children, spouses, and other loved
ones. Additionally, methamphetamine production

exposes anyone near the process to toxic chemicals and the risk of explosion.

My Administration is committed to fighting the spread of methamphetamine abuse throughout our country. While the number of teens who have tried this deadly drug and the number of people testing positive for methamphetamine in the workplace have decreased in recent years, methamphetamine use is still a dangerous public health problem. In the Synthetic Drug Control Strategy released earlier this year, my Administration set goals of a 15 percent decrease in methamphetamine use and 25 percent reduction in domestic methamphetamine labs over the next 3 years. To help reach these objectives, my proposed 2007 budget includes $25 million to help ensure that Americans have access to effective methamphetamine abuse recovery services and programs. Earlier this year, I also signed into law the Combat Methamphetamine Epidemic Act of 2005, which makes manufacturing the drug more difficult and imposes tougher penalties on those who smuggle or sell it.

The struggle against methamphetamine is a national, State, and local effort. By working together, we can build a stronger, healthier America for generations to come.

NOW, THEREFORE, I, GEORGE W. BUSH, President of the United States of America, by virtue of the authority vested in me by the Constitution and laws of the United States, do hereby proclaim November 30, 2006, as National Methamphetamine Awareness Day. I call upon the people of the United States to observe this day with appropriate programs and activities.

IN WITNESS WHEREOF, I have hereunto set my hand this twenty-seventh day of November, in the year of our Lord two thousand six, and of the Independence of the United States of America the two hundred and thirty-first.

GEORGE W. BUSH ●

THE SHAPE OF SPEED TO COME

"A POPPY FLOWERS IN ASIA, AND A JUNKIE DIES IN NEW York. Coca leaves bend in a Peruvian sunshower as bullets hail down on a dealer in Miami. A kitchen chemist brews a designer drug as disease eats away a user's brain. A physician injects himself with a painkiller as a mother gives birth to an addicted baby. At work and at play people use uppers and downers, even drugs that seem to turn them upside down, while governments search for direction in controlling an overwhelming number of chemical recreations that keep flowing through our lives and bodies politic. These scenes from the modern drug world are neither new nor unique events in history. Old World explorers, medieval herbalists, ancient Greeks, Neolithic shamans, beasts, and bugs everywhere have had accidental or intentional encounters with drugs."

—Ronald K. Siegel Ph.D., *Intoxication* (Dutton 1989)

In the fullness of history, all the different varieties of speed may have been products of the twentieth century, even though they are still around nearly a decade into the twenty-first, and show no sign of waning. Speed is too much of a reflection of its time. The twentieth century was an era of acceleration. Humanity went from its first powered flight to a moon landing in less than 70 years. Two atomic weapons were deliberately detonated over inhabited cities, while other cities were turned into unstoppable firestorms by tons of conventional explosives dropped from high-flying aircraft. Millions died in two devastating world wars, and millions more in smaller wars, insurrections, and ethnic cleansings. We have seen the computer grow from a mechanical adding machine to an entity so powerful and omnipresent that speculation is now possible about the likelihood of machines merging identities with humanity. The event of rock & roll added a frenetic thrashing drive to the world's entertainment, and television warped the world's perception. The twentieth century was an era of massive overreaching that culminated in us pushing our planet to the very edge of environmental catastrophe, as melting icecaps change the course of the ocean tides.

The twentieth century was also a time of scarcely believable greed and all too grandiose dreams. The developed nations of the West demanded more and more, and we grew furious if TV commercials reneged on their promises and we couldn't instantly have it all. The West grew fat even as famines decimated developing nations. We burned energy as if there was no tomorrow, and in so doing, made tomorrow considerably more problematic. And this was where speed found its place, introducing itself to greedy dreams on all levels of twentieth-century culture with seductive assurances of free additional energy, enhancing stamina that enabled users to keep going like the bunny in battery commercial, and feel a euphoric omnipotence as the need to eat, sleep, or even feel anything unwontedly profound were removed by the insulating effects of amphetamine. One could even lose radical weight with no effort of will, and become fashionably slim.

Adolf Hitler's doctor shot him up with cocktails of speed and the devil only knew what else, as he designed the blitzkrieg, in his greed for the absolute power he believed would enable him to annex the entire planet for his master race, and organized the deaths of tens of millions. Jack Kennedy's doctor shot him up with similar hellish cocktails, but during the Cuba missile crisis, Kennedy was able to steer a course through the nuclear minefield of mutually assured destruction, save the lives of hundreds of millions, and set America on the course for that first moment on the moon, and inspire aspirations to the mastery of space and the universe. The Beatles popped pills from a German pharmacy, and played endless, hour on/hour off shows to drunken sailors and their whores, in pimp-infested cellars on Hamburg's red-light Reeperbahn, while dreaming of the kind of rock & roll fame only achieved by Elvis Presley, who had swallowed his mother's diet pills while attempting to understand why fate had dealt him such a bizarre hand of cards, and why so many millions of people wanted a part of him. Hugh Hefner popped pills and turned the airbrushed nudity of invitingly contorted playmates into a twentieth century institution, and although he supposedly rarely slept in his heyday, he ran a quasi-erotic empire from his circular bed.

The honeymoon promises of speed became part of the underpinnings of many of the grand illusions and monstrous debacles of the time. The way in which both the Nazi and Imperial Japanese war machines placed a major reliance on the drug to provide them with indefatigable storm troopers, and kamikazes who didn't fear death. Amphetamines have woven a hidden but ubiquitous thread through the entire history of the twentieth century and have been a factor in some of its most chaotic episodes. In many ways the story of amphetamine itself, and the course followed by the typical speedfreak are natural parallels. Both start with a sense of euphoria, an optimistic energy that a solution has been found, and that all things are possible. Speed promises something for nothing and tears down normal boundaries, but as time passes, a form of entropy begins to take its toll, and circumstances start to appear less and less rational.

When Benzedrine first went on sale in the 1930s, it was without too much fanfare, but the drug was quickly adopted on multiple levels of society. Its potential to give an instant boost appealed to a variety of people in a whole range of occupations. Even before World War II, intimations were already being noticed that maybe speed wasn't quite the wonder drug of first impression. More and more had to be consumed to achieve the same result. The drug became too central to the lives of those using it, and some found it hard to decide if they were speeding to live, or living to speed. The realization gradually dawned that it was perhaps an illusion that one could get something for nothing, and that ultimately a price would have to be paid. Women who used speed to make them witty and vivacious, and to gain the perfect figure were the first to realize that slim and tireless could all too easily turn into emaciated and insane. Athletes who used the drug to give them an edge found that not only was the supposed edge illusionary and easily blunted, but that their overall game began to disintegrate. Lovers who took speed for the sexual rush found that it was a hit and miss blessing, and tended to distort the true nature of the underlying relationship.

Artists who made amphetamine central to their creativity found that speed was also becoming central to their art and actually limiting its potential, or, as in the case of director and choreographer Bob Fosse, if they were able to maintain the furious pace permitted by taking more and more of the drug, and corral all the random ideas that came with it, their bodies gave out on them. Speed is a highly narcissistic drug, artificially inflating the sense of self as the intrusion of external stimuli is progressively reduced. In an inspired piece of narcissism, Fosse made the film *All That Jazz* as a quasi-autobiography, and a frighteningly accurate prophecy of his own heart attack and death. The audience is shown Roy Scheider as Fosse, simultaneously editing a major motion picture, casting and directing a Broadway show, and carrying on disastrous affairs with a number of women. He smokes cigarettes in the shower, he swallows Dexedrine, and even though his mind drifts into eerie silences, he refuses to halt his headlong charge. In the end his heart gives out and he dies on the operating table. His death is played as an elaborate singing/dancing production number set to the Everly Brothers' tune "Bye

Bye Love"—with it's the ominous line at the end the cho-
rus, "I think I'm gonna die."

Although Bob Fosse's real life was undoubtedly shortened by his frenzied use of speed to keep up with an impossible workload, a rule does emerge that speedfreaks
with a mission, a purpose, or an occupation tend to handle
the drug better than those without. Long distance truckers
and other traditional amphetamine users show less damage
from speed than kids getting out of their minds on crank
while staring into a TV, playing video games, or simply
vibrating to the latest in thrash metal. The essential difference between the rock & rollers of the 1960s and 1970s,
and the tweakers of the 1990s and twenty-first century is
that the rockers—not only The Beatles, The Who, and The
Clash, but many, many, more—used the drug as a means
to an end rather than an end in itself. The question the
Montana Meth Project fails to address is that, if an unreal
percentage of young people in Montana are using crystal
meth, and showing signs of damage, maybe there's something wrong with Montana. If crystal meth is the strongest
and most satisfying stimulant they can find, their hori-
zons have to be depressingly narrow, and other sources of
stimulation few and far between.

Speed creates a restless impatience that, unless channelled, can simply turn on the user and make itself the sole
fixation of his and her life. The drug takes over like an all
consuming obsession that seems preferable to some dead-
end, minimum-wage job. A barrage of media promotion,
both above and below the radar, attempts to program adolescents to be passive consumers. Discontent and natural
youth rebellion, if they haven't already been dulled and

distorted by the Ritalin and Adderall prescribed for them in school, is channelled into the electronic pseudo-aggression of *Grand Theft Auto*. For a kid in these circumstances, a first speed encounter must feel like revelation of previously undreamed of depth. A myriad of illusions present themselves, but the truth is that they remain illusions.

The trouble really starts when the speedfreak discovers, through long days and jagged sleepless nights, that a life wholly based on the consumption of crystal meth is, in reality, mind-snappingly boring. It becomes a cycle of running franticly with the drug or desperately crashing, while the total disorganization of the speedfreak's grasshopper thought processes, and the criminal milieu in which the illegality of meth forces him or her to exist, is the source of a multitude of nagging fears and paranoia. Inevitably a full divorce from reality will come in the form of some full blown psychotic episode. Most of the time this tearing of the emotional fabric will not manifest itself in anything more than shaking, alone in a room, wide-eyed and temporarily lost to everything rational, or going out on the street and screaming to the sun, moon or an invisible friend, a variation of "I'm mad as hell and I'm not going to take it anymore." Unless blind luck somehow holds, the freaker will be spotted up by the police, arrested, and become one more statistic in the methedrine-related crime figures.

Only the truly exceptional cases of amphetamine psychosis—like the terminally demented speedfreak in San Diego who stole the Abrams tank, went on his car-crushing, solo destruction derby, and was shot by the cops for his trouble—make it onto the TV news. A character like

Andrew Cunanan, the gay, speedfreak killer of the ultra-successful fashion designer Gianni Versace, is the exception rather than the rule. The three-month, cross-country killing spree that Cunanan undertook in the summer of 1997 has been frequently cited as a "typical" result of long-term methamphetamine use. Nothing is typical about Cunanan's homicidal drive to Florida during which he murdered two former lovers, Jeffrey Trail and David Madson, and also Lee Miglin, a Chicago real estate millionaire, and the unfortunate William Reese, who Cunanan killed simply to steal his truck as a replacement vehicle.

After Cunanan stalked and killed Versace, pumping two shots into the back of the designer's head as he entered his mansion home, he holed up on a Florida houseboat, and finally killed himself with a single shot in the mouth. All analysis of his behavior were therefore made postmortem, without any questioning or study of Cunanan's motivation or mindset, or any other mental disorders from which he might have suffered. The point was repeatedly made at the time that Cunanan appeared to take an unholy delight in killing, and that he was driven by an enduring and inescapable rage. He wrapped one victim's head in duct tape, before stabbing him in the chest with pruning sheers, beating him, and cutting his throat with a hack saw. Not content with all of that, Cunanan repeatedly drove over the body until it was pulped. To attribute all this to the effects of methamphetamine is both implausible and shortsighted, in that it is so simplistic it adds nothing to our understanding of future spree killers.

Cunanan biographer Maureen Orth quotes a supposed acquaintance of the killer called Vance Coukoulis in her 1999 book *Vulgar Favors*, but in so doing, she plays not only into the demonization of speed-users, but also into a serious level of homophobia: "It's a sex drug, and all it does is just heighten your whole sexual feeling about a million times." He also adds that, "It makes you think about sex 24 hours a day. The whole system's become so promiscuous it's frightening. I believed in the devil after I got involved with the gay society and crystal meth, and then I realized evil existed in human nature and that human nature can be of good or of evil, and I really believe in evil now. Period. And I believe an evil spirit can overtake people, and I believe that's what happened to Andrew. He changed through the use of that drug."

To anthropomorphize a chemical and then make it fully responsible for an episode of homicidal psychosis is simply sensationalism at its worst. Plus, it totally matches the most luridly cynical drug warrior propaganda, and clouds any real truth about why Cunanan did what he did. It overlooks how the repeated and seemingly unstoppable crystal meth epidemics that regularly sweep the country are actually created by the blind, single-mindedness, and poor long-term planning by the DEA, and all the other branches of federal and local law enforcement waging the War On Drugs. Maybe all that stands repeating is that the War on Drugs has been waged for more than 70 years, and the mess created by recreational drug use while it remains outlawed but unchecked and unregulated, grows more debilitating and chaotic each year and each decade.

One day, sooner or later, the War On Drugs will end. All indications are that the end will come later rather than sooner, but nothing so farcically unworkable can survive forever. Although, from today's perspective, any cessation of these domestic hostilities may look impossible when one considers the number and size of the vested interests in what one wag dubbed the "drug enforcement industry," and the vast corporate profits that are made on the back of the status quo from everything from the supply of elaborate high-tech equipment to cops and agents, to outsourced private prisons. The United States has the dubious honor of being the worlds biggest jailer, with the highest per capita prison population of any country—some 738 per 100,000 of its citizens. During 2006 the total federal, state, and local adult correctional population rose to over 7.2 million, which is about 3.2 percent of the US adult population, or one in every 31 adults. Although only one quarter of prison inmates have been convicted of drug offences, estimates of those in jail for *drug-related* crimes runs as high as a massive 80 percent of the entire prison population. Combine these prison numbers with the figures for drug related deaths, the cumulated billions spent on the Drug War, and its overall ineffectiveness, and if only to retain one's sanity, the hope has to be that the American people eventually elect an administration that has the courage to heed the Drug Policy Alliance's basic tenets of harm reduction—"There has never been, is not now, and never will be a drug-free society. Harm reduction approach acknowledges that there is no ultimate solution to the problem of drugs in a free society, and that many different interventions may work. Those interventions should be based on science, compassion, health and human rights."

Despite all the continuing furor over methamphetamine, it is likely, whether the War On Drugs continues or not, that the current crank epidemic will tail off, and although speed will probably be with us in any foreseeable future, it will not be grabbing the same screaming headlines. Drug panics would appear to be subject to a kind of natural entropy and will fade away of their own accord. In the latter half of the 1970s, angel dust—the popular name for the animal tranquilizer PCP—was public enemy number one among illegal drugs. At the time, the media couldn't get enough of stories about angel dust users being overwhelmed by nightmare hallucinations and fighting off police with the strength of 10, but by the mid-to-late 1980s, angel dust was forgotten, and crack cocaine had taken its place as the major source of drug panic—even though the CIA and the Iran-Contra conspiracy was assisting its spread in major cities like Los Angeles.

This is not to say that crack and angel dust vanished from the face of the Earth. They simply became another drug in the market place. Like so much else in contemporary society, drug use is subject to the fluctuations of fad and fashion. A media drug panic indicates that the same drug is also enjoying a street level vogue, but vogues tend to be short-lived and fickle. Peripheral users are temporarily drawn to the drug, but for many, the novelty soon wears off, and they move on to other highs. Deaths occur among the hardcore, others are busted and imprisoned, some seek cures, and still more simply give up. The media can also prove as fickle as fashion, and drug panic stories quickly grow tired. Once out of the spotlight, a drug epidemic is frequently revealed not to be as bad as was first imagined, as soon as its free of the shock-horror items on TV news. The very same thing could happen with crystal meth. While speed presents an unquestionably serious problem, especially in suburban and rural areas, there is a reasonable chance that many of the current generation of Middle American speeds freaks will grow out of their self-destructive obsession. The chances will improve greatly, if instead of demonizing these people as meth monsters, they are given a shot at an education, and more positive choices of ways to spend their time and lives.

We are still in the first decade of the twenty-first century, and the future is not easy to predict. Planet Earth currently holds out little cause for optimism, but one thing is for sure. Things will change, and very little is going to stay the same. Methamphetamine may have actually bottomed out with these crystal meth epidemics. All the promise once looked for in speed has become history, and now, even to the perception of other parts of the drug culture, it is the sole province of hopeless, Jerry Springer, untutored trailer trash. (While we forget that thousands of anonymous and outwardly normal folk take a hit of speed to help them get through the day without anyone noticing.) For all we know, another decade may see a new drug come out of nowhere, and revolutionize our ideas of intoxication to the same degree that acid did in the 1960s, when acidheads seemed little short of an alien invasion to the generation that looked for relief in dry martinis. Speed may already be obsolete, except we have nothing quite yet to replace it.

If the day ever came when the drug warriors finally folded their tents and gave up their impossible dream of a drug-free nation, the world would be open to the pharmaceutical corporations actually designing a menu of safe intoxicants that could allow people to get high without the risk of mental, physical, or legal damage. Our culture is already awash in medication. We are sold Prozac and Ativan to take the edge off depression, Viagra as a chemical sex aid, and Ambien or Lunestra to help us sleep. We have specific drugs for twitchy legs and irritable bowels. Advertisements for them crowd the commercial spots on prime time TV selling us cures for ailments we didn't know existed until they told us about them, and also list the side effects of the cure. Electronics now take such massive strides that it's possible, within little more than a generation, that direct cortical stimuli or even microscopic nanobots working directly on the receptors and the pleasure centers of the brain might make the ingesting of crude chemicals like amphetamine, alcohol, or even acid, a piece of history quite as quaint as the Victorian taste for opium-based remedies and tinctures.

Even without some science fiction revolution in the very real human need for regular intoxication, the patterns of our drug use in the future will inevitably change, and so will the drugs themselves. New factors will be introduced, and the older needs will be met by other means, or simply fall by the wayside. We have looked at the strange evolution of amphetamine in the twentieth century, from Benzedrine inhalers to super labs, and the way that evolution has impacted all levels of society, from a president in the White House to uneducated, rural teenagers. That this very rapid metamorphosis will suddenly stop can hardly be plausible. So far, it has occurred every time new pressures come to bear, and shows no indication of doing otherwise. One thing we can certainly count on in the twenty-first century is that we will see a multitude of new and unique pressures. Like it or not, speedfreaks have lived through and contributed to what amounts to a not insignificant historical saga. They are still with us and show no signs of stumbling away or taking their drugs with them. The face of the future speedfreak will be revealed in the fullness of time, and the only guarantee is that it probably won't be what we expect, because the speed of the future will wholly depend on one single factor.

How crazy do future generations want to be? ●

Speed-Speed-Speedfreak
© 2010 by Mick Farren and Feral House
All rights reserved.

A Feral House Book

Feral House
1240 W. Sims Way Suite 124
Port Townsend WA 98368

www.FeralHouse.com

ISBN: 978-1-932595-82-6

10 9 8 7 6 5 4 3 2 1

printed in China

Cover and interior design by Bill Smith